Super Tasty Mediterranean Cookbook

Fit and Healthy Recipes

For Busy People

Ben Cooper

Table of contents

Classic Greek Salad
Preparation Time: 15 minutes
Cooking Time: 0 minutes
Servings: 6

Ingredients:

6 large firm tomatoes, quartered
20 Greek black olives
½ lb. Greek feta cheese, cut into small cubes
½ head of escarole, shredded
3 tbsp. red wine vinegar
¼ cup extra-virgin olive oil
1 tbsp. dried oregano
½ English cucumber, peeled, seeded, and thinly sliced
2 cloves fresh garlic, finely minced
½ red onion, sliced
1 medium red bell pepper, seeded and sliced
¼ cup freshly chopped Italian parsley Salt and freshly
ground pepper to taste

Directions:

1.Take out a large bowl and add vinegar, oregano, olive
oil, and garlic. Add salt and pepper to taste. Set aside
the bowl.

2.In another large bowl, add onion, tomatoes, escarole,
cucumber, bell pepper, and cheese and mix them well.

3.Take the vinegar mixture and pour it over the salad in
the second bowl.

4.Top the salad with olives and parsley.

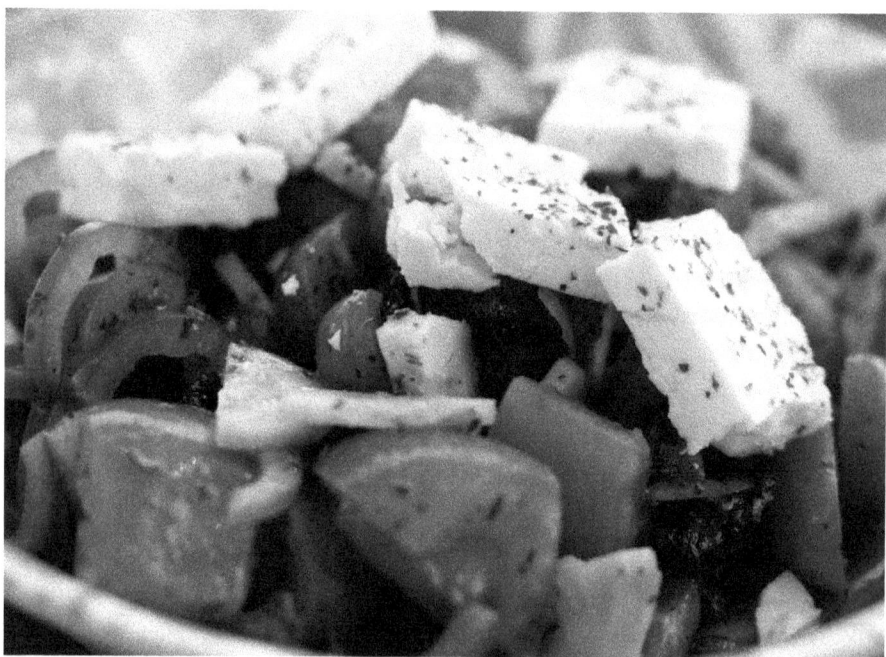

North African Zucchini Salad

Preparation Time: 10 minutes

Cooking Time: 0 minutes

Servings: 4

Ingredients:

1 lb. firm green zucchini, thinly sliced
½ tsp. ground cumin
2 cloves fresh garlic, finely minced Juice from
1 large lemon
1 tbsp. extra-virgin olive oil
1½ tbsp. plain low-fat yogurt Crumbled feta cheese
Finely chopped parsley for garnish
Salt and freshly ground pepper to taste

Directions:

1. Add the zucchini into a large saucepan and steam it for about 2-5 minutes, or until it becomes tender and crispy. Place the zucchini under cold water and drain well.

2.Take out a large bowl and mix cumin, olive oil, lemon juice, garlic, and yogurt. Add salt and pepper to taste.

3.Add the zucchini into the mixture in the bowl and toss gently.

4.Serve with feta cheese and parsley as garnish.

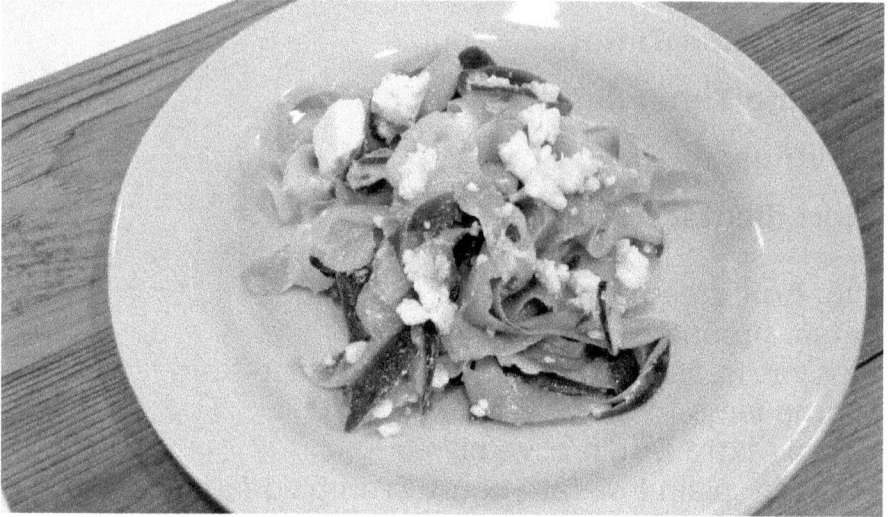

Tunisian Style Carrot Salad

Preparation Time: 15 minutes

Cooking Time: 0 minutes

Servings: 6

Ingredients:

10 medium carrots, peeled and sliced
1 cup crumbled feta cheese, divided
2 tsp. caraway seed
¼ cup extra-virgin olive oil
6 tbsp. apple cider vinegar
5 tsp. freshly minced garlic
1 tbsp. Harissa paste (choose the level of heat based on your preference)
20 pitted Kalamata olives, reserving some for garnish
Salt to taste

Directions:

1.Take out a medium saucepan and place it on medium heat. Fill it with water and add the carrots. Cook carrots until tender. Drain and cool the carrots under cold water. Drain again to remove any excess water.

2.Take out a large bowl and place the carrots in them.

3.Take out a mortar and combine salt, garlic, and caraway seeds. Grind them until they form a paste. Otherwise, you can also use a small bowl, preferably one not made out of glass for grind.

4.The final option would be to toss the ingredients into a blender and pulse them.

5.Add vinegar and Harissa into the bowl with the carrots and mix them well.

6.Use a large spoon and mash the carrots. Add the garlic mixture into the carrot and mix again until they have all blended well. Add the olive oil and mix again.

7Finally, add about ½ the feta cheese and all the olives and mix well again.

8.Take out a large bowl and add the salad to it. Top it with the remaining feta cheese.

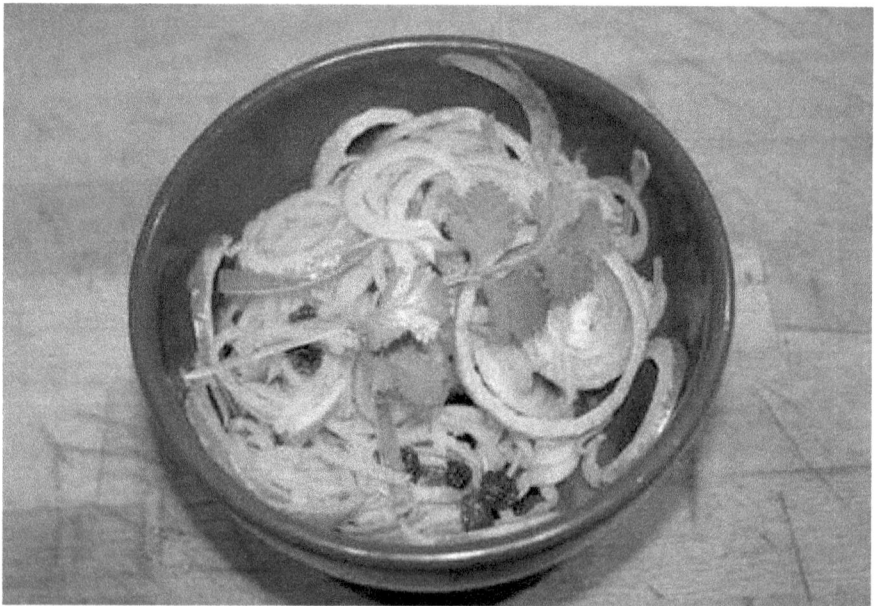

Caesar Salad

Preparation Time: 5 minutes
Cooking Time: 0 minutes
Servings: 6

Ingredients:

10 small pitted black olives, chopped
1-2 bunches romaine lettuce, cleaned and torn in pieces
2 tsp. lemon juice
2½ tsp. balsamic vinegar
½ cup grated parmesan cheese
½ cup nonfat plain yogurt
1 tsp. worcestershire sauce
½ tsp. anchovy paste
2 cloves freshly minced garlic

Directions:

1.Take out a large bowl and place romaine lettuce in it.

2.Take out your blended and add mix lemon juice, yogurt, garlic, anchovy paste, vinegar, worcestershire sauce, and ¼ cup parmesan cheese. Mix all the ingredients well until they are smooth.

3.Pour the yogurt mixture over the lettuce and toss lightly.

4.Top the salad with the remaining parmesan cheese.

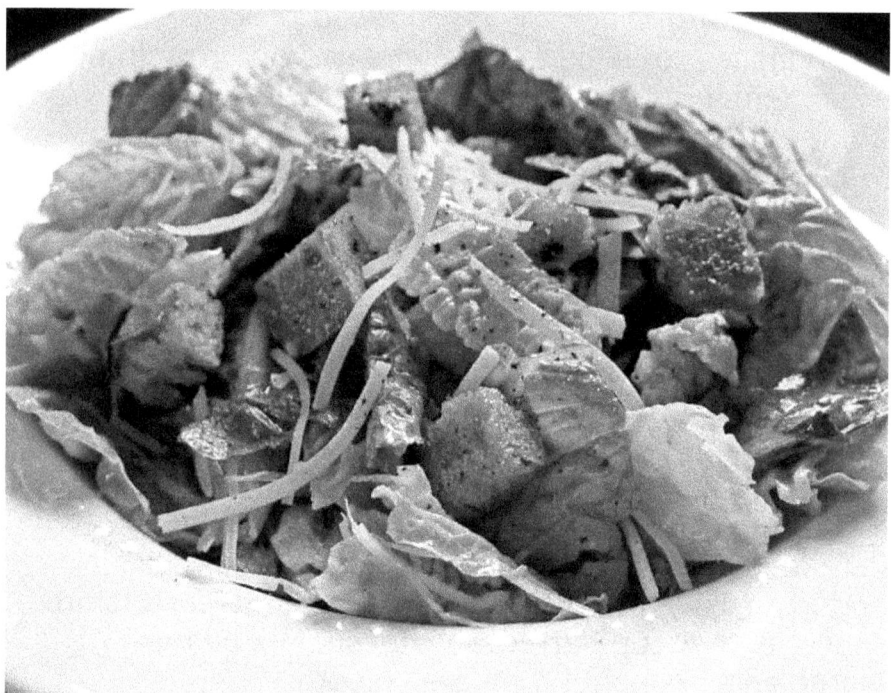

Cress and Tangerine Salad

Preparation Time: 15 minutes

Cooking Time: 0 minutes

Servings: 4

Ingredients:
4 large sweet tangerines
¼ cup extra-virgin olive oil
2 large bunches watercress, washed and stems removed Juice from
1 fresh lemon
10 cherry tomatoes, halved
16 pitted Kalamata olives
Sea salt and freshly ground pepper to taste

Directions:

1.Take the tangerines and peel them into a medium-sized bowl. Make sure that you remove any pits and squeeze the sections. You should have around ¼ cup of tangerine juice. Set sections aside.

2.Take a large bowl and add lemon juice, tangerine juice, and olive oil. Mix them and add salt and pepper for flavor, if you prefer.

3. Use paper towels to pat the cress dry. Add watercress, tomatoes, and olives to the bowl containing the tangerine sections (not to be confused with the bowl containing tangerine juice). Toss them lightly.

4.Pour the tangerine juice mixture on top. Mix well and serve.

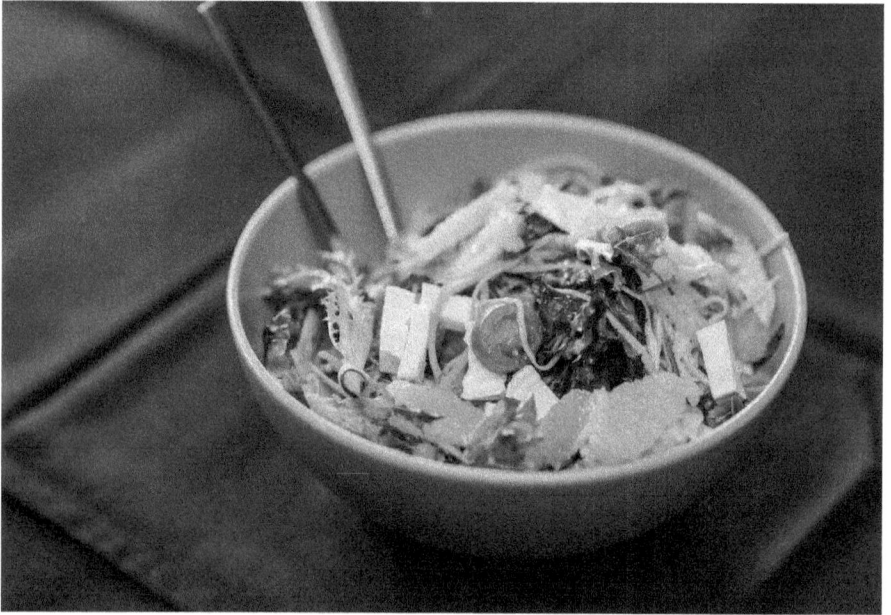

Prosciutto and Figs Salad

Preparation Time: 10 minutes

Cooking Time: 0 minutes

Servings: 4

Ingredients:

110-12-oz. package fresh baby spinach
1 small hot red chili pepper, finely diced
1 carton figs, stems removed and quartered
½ cup walnuts, coarsely chopped
1 tbsp. fresh orange juice
1 tbsp. honey
4 slices prosciutto, cut into strips
Shaved parmesan cheese for garnish

Directions:

1.Take your spinach and divide them into 4 equal portions. Each portion should be on a separate plate and will act as a base. Add quartered prosciutto, figs, and walnuts on each spinach as toppings.

2.For the dressing, take a small bowl and add honey, orange juice, and diced pepper. Add the mixture over the salad.

3.Finally, toss the salad lightly and use parmesan cheese for the garnish.

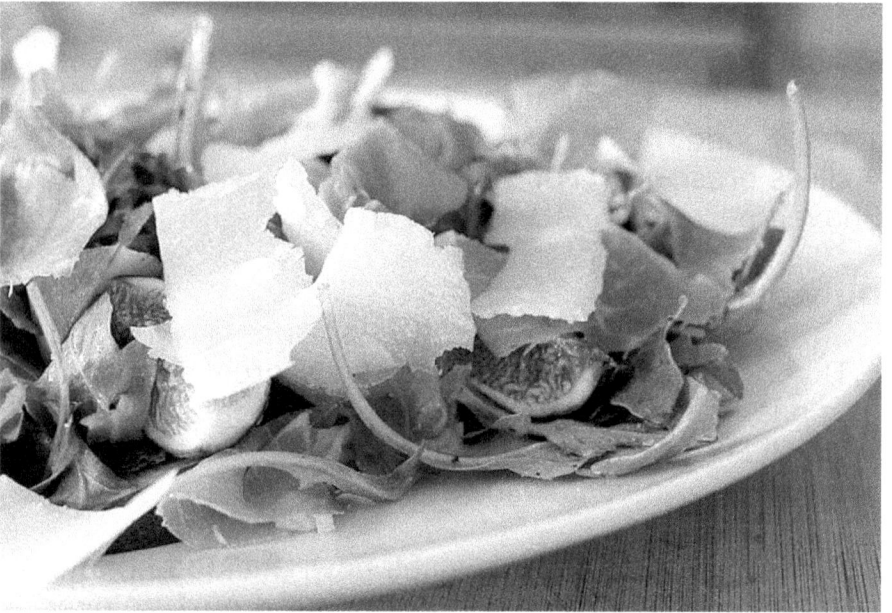

Garden Vegetables and Chickpeas Salad

Preparation Time: 10 minutes

Cooking Time: 0 minutes

Servings: 4

Ingredients:

2 tbsp. freshly squeezed lemon juice
1/8 tsp. freshly ground pepper
1 cup cubed part-skim mozzarella cheese
1 tbsp. fresh basil leaf, snipped
1 (15-oz.) can chickpeas, rinsed and well drained
2 cups coarsely chopped fresh broccoli
2 cloves fresh garlic, finely minced
½ cup sliced fresh carrots
1 7½-oz. can diced tomatoes, undrained

Directions:

1.Use a large bowl and add garlic, basil, lemon juice, and ground pepper. Mix them well.

2.Add the chickpeas, carrots, tomatoes with juice, broccoli, and mozzarella cheese. Toos all the ingredients well.

3.You can serve immediately, or you can keep it refrigerated overnight.

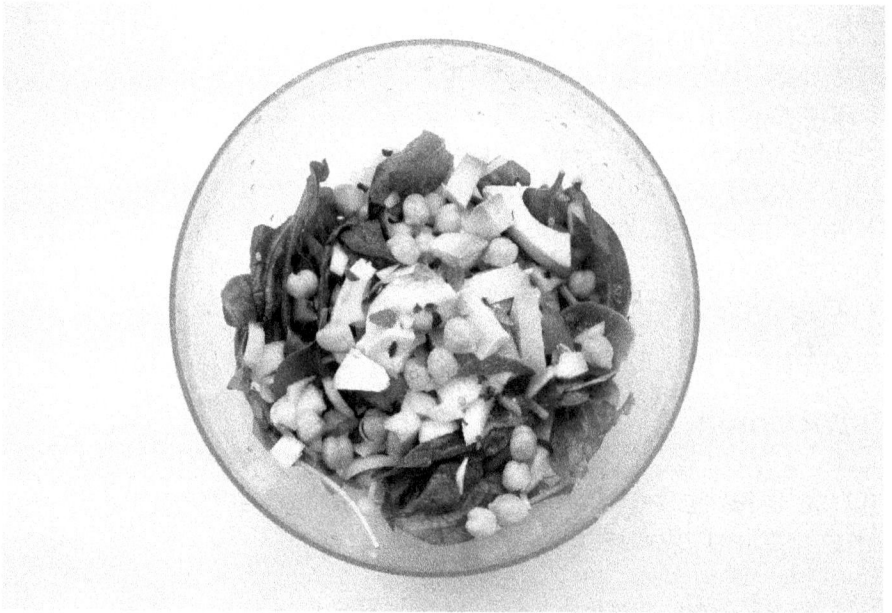

Peppered Watercress Salad

Preparation Time: 5 minutes

Cooking Time: 0 minutes

Servings: 4

Ingredients:

2 tsp. champagne vinegar
2 bunches (about 8 cups) watercress, rinsed and rough stems removed
2 tbsp. extra-virgin olive oil
Salt and freshly ground pepper to taste

Directions:

1.Drain the watercress properly.

2.Take out a small bowl and then add salt, pepper, vinegar, and olive oil. Mix them well together.

3.Transfer the watercress to a bowl. Add the vinegar mixture into it and toss well.

4.Serve immediately.

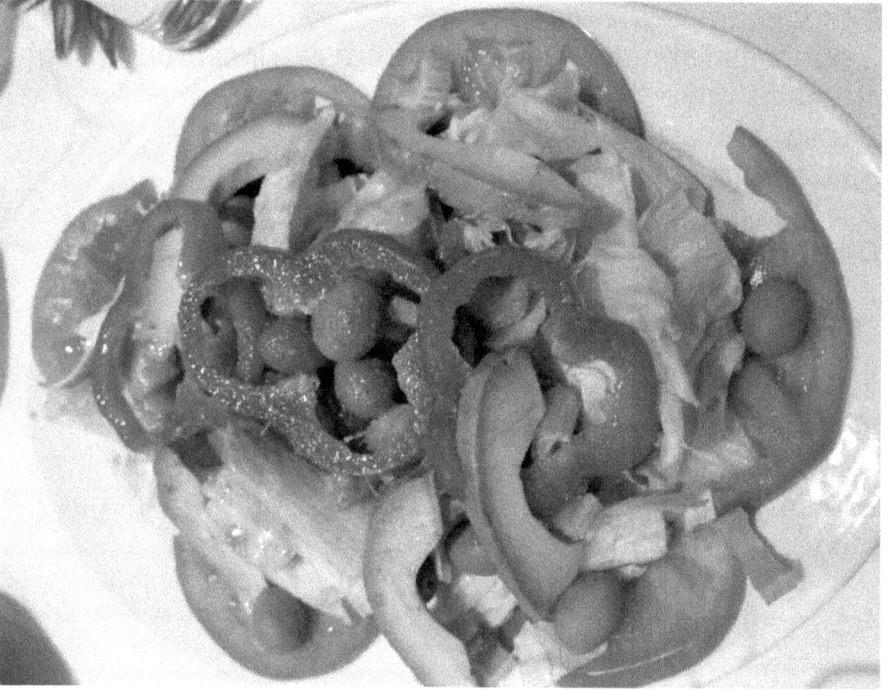

Baked egg with cheddar and beef

Preparation time: 20 minutes
Cooking time: 20 minutes
Servings: 6

Ingredients:

6 eggs
1 lb beef
1 chopped green pepper
Salt to taste
Pepper to taste
1 cup green beans Cream of mushroom soup
1/2 cup shredded cheddar cheese
1 cup almond milk
1 tbsp vegetable oil
1 cup mushrooms
1 tsp onion powder
2 tbsp cornstarch
1/2 tsp salt

Directions:

1.Cook beef with beans and bell pepper.

2.Crack eggs and cook for five minutes.

3.Transfer the beef to the casserole and pour mushroom soup and toss.

4.Bake in a preheated oven at 350 degrees for 20 minutes. Cream of Mushroom Soup

5.Blend all the items of mushroom soup in the blender.

6.Boil the mixture and simmer it for 12 minutes.

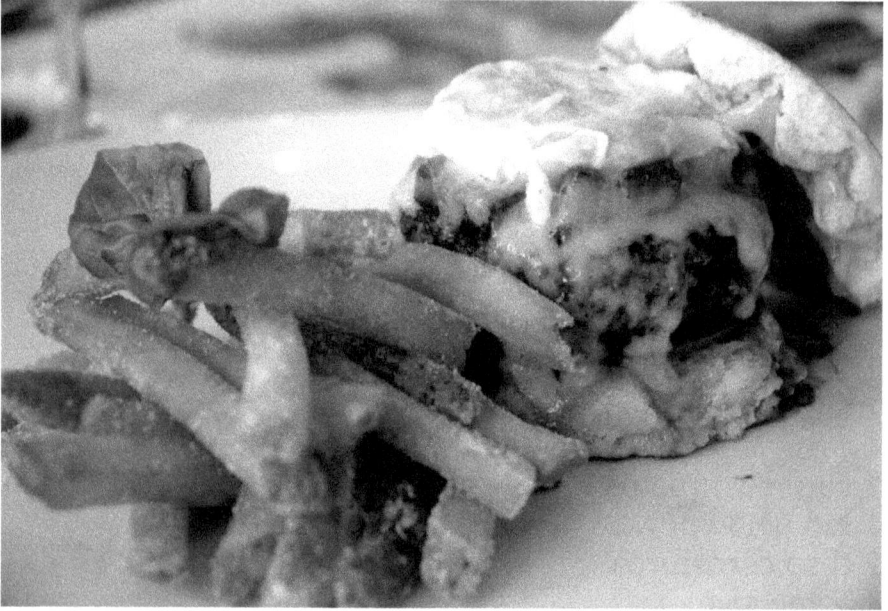

Heavenly egg bake with pancakes

Preparation time: 15 minutes
Cooking time: 25 minutes
Servings: 8

Ingredients:

2 cups baking mix
2 cups shredded Cheddar cheese
1 cup milk
5 tbsp maple syrup
2 eggs
1.5 tbsp white sugar
12 slices cooked bacon

Directions:

1.Mix all the ingredients in a bowl and bake in a preheated oven at 350 degrees for 25 minutes.

2.Top with cheese and bacon and bake for five more minutes.

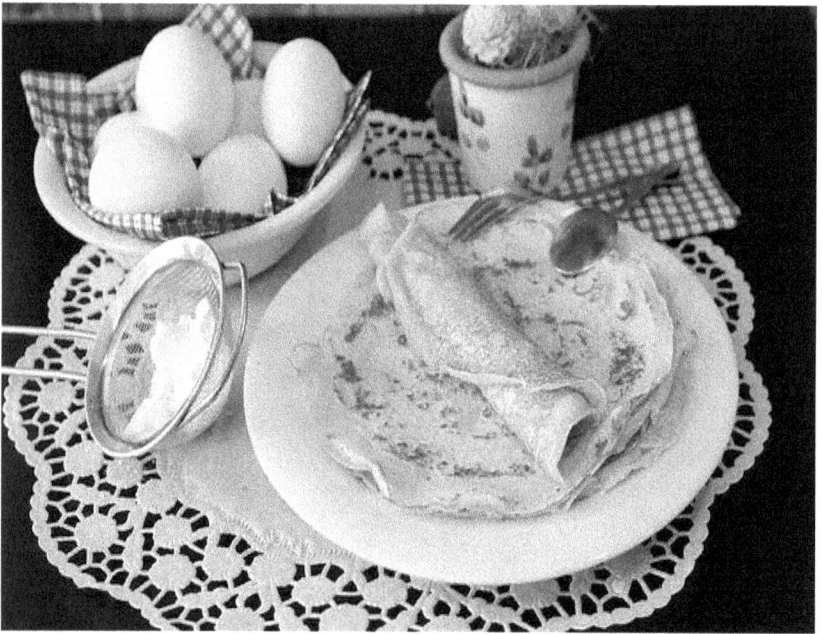

Coffee with butter

Preparation time: 5 minutes
Cooking time: 5 minutes
Servings: 1

Ingredients:
1 cup hot coffee
2 tbsp butter
1 tbsp coconut oil

Directions:

1.Combine all the items in a blender and serve.

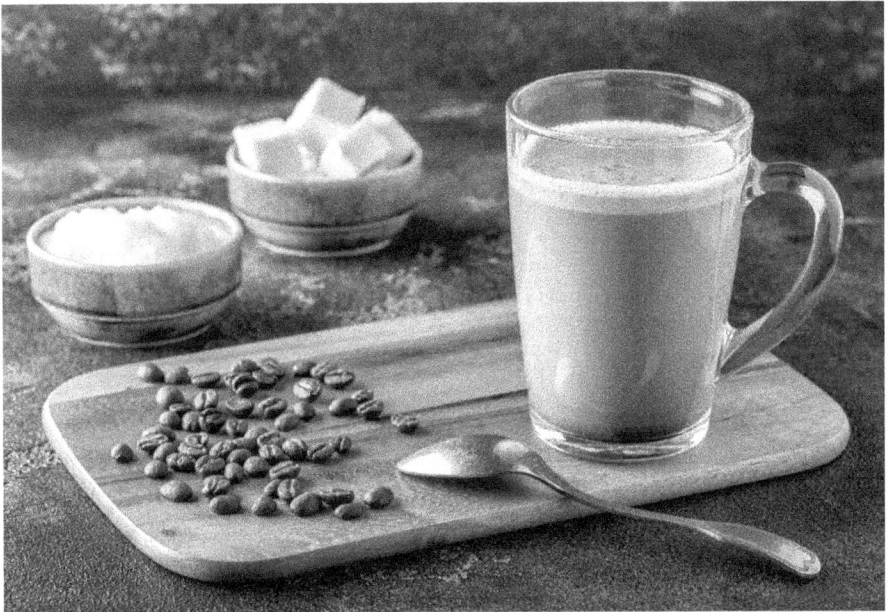

Creamy Cheese Pancake

Preparation time: 2 minutes
Cooking time: 6 minutes
Servings: 4

Ingredients:

1 lb sea scallops
4 thyme
Salt to taste
Black pepper to taste
2 tbsp butter
2 lemons
1 tbsp olive oil

Directions:

1.Cook scallops for five minutes over a high flame in a skillet.

2.Stir in herbs and cook in butter for six minutes.

3.Squeeze lemon juice and serve.

Persimmon toast with cream

Preparation time: 5 minutes
Cooking time: 0 minutes
Servings: 1

Ingredients:

1 sliced bread
1 Sour cream
1/2 Persimmon
1 Cinnamon
1 Granulated sugar

Directions:

1.Place cream over bread and lay persimmon slices.

2.Drizzle sugar and cinnamon.

3.Bake in preheated oven for five minutes at 250 degrees

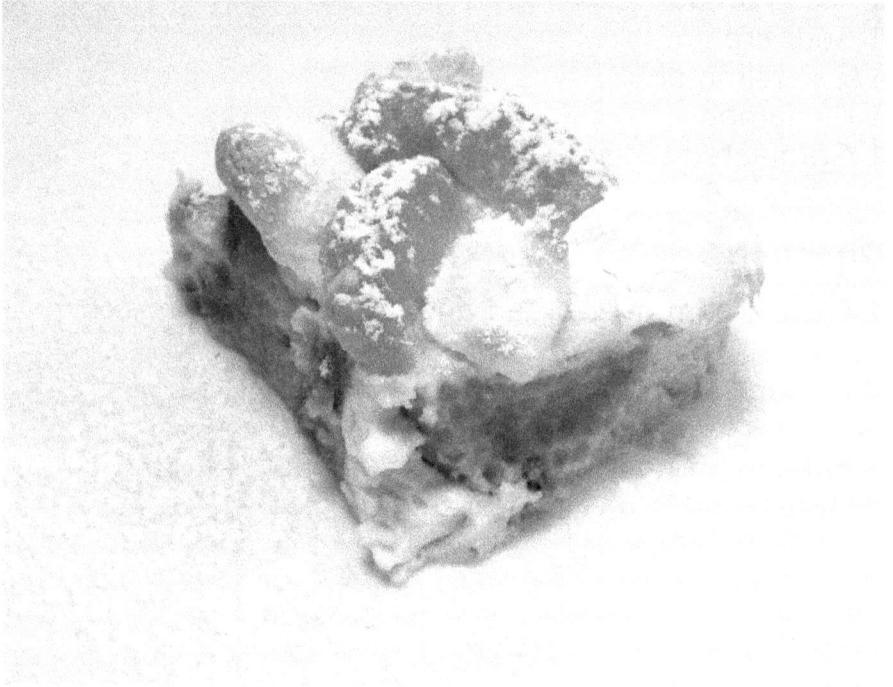

Tofu with mushrooms

Preparation time: 25 minutes
Cooking time: 17 minutes
Servings: 4

Ingredients:

Pepper to taste
1 tbsp sweetener
1 tbsp Hoisin sauce
14 oz tofu
5 tbsp soy sauce
1 lb Cremini mushrooms
1 pinch of red color
1 tbsp rice vinegar
2 tsp peanut oil
3 sliced ginger
1 tsp sesame oil
3 sliced garlic cloves
1/2 cup sliced green onions

Directions:

1.Marinate tofu with a mixture of vinegar, pepper, soy sauce, and sesame oil in a bowl.

2.Drain tofu after 30 minutes of marination.

3.Add agav to the marination mixture.

4.Sauté ginger and garlic in heated oil over medium flame.

5.Mix in tofu and cook for ten minutes.

6.After seven minutes, take out tofu and set aside.

7.Pour oil and add mushrooms and cook for five more minutes.

8.Again put tofu in the pan and cook.

9.Pour in sauce mixture and reduce the flame and cook for five minutes.

10.Stir in onions and cook for two minutes.

11.Serve and enjoy it.

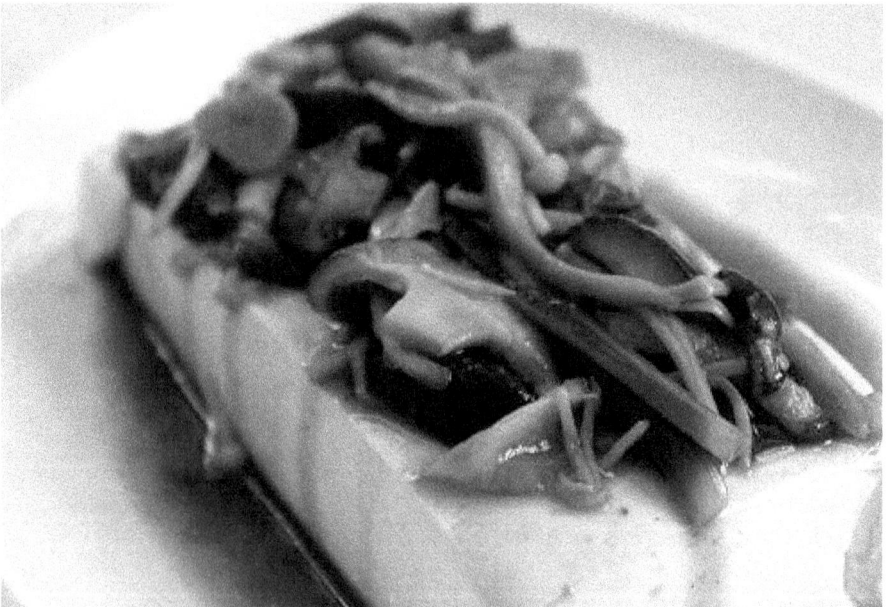

Ham spinach ballet

Preparation time: 10 minutes
Cooking time: 22 minutes
Servings: 6

Ingredients:

1/2 cup ham
1/4 tsp seasoned salt
1/2 tsp dry mustard
1.5 cups spinach
2 tbsp olive oil
8 eggs
1/4 cup half and half
1/2 pound potatoes
2 green onions sliced
1/4 tsp black pepper
1/2 cup cheddar cheese divided

Directions:

1.Preheat the oven up to 400°F.

2.Heat olive oil in a skillet. Add potatoes & water. Season with salt & pepper

3.Now stir, Cover & cook (10-15 min) until softened.

4.Stir in ham, green & spinach along with onions until hot & spinach is wilted.

5.Take a bowl combine egg, dry mustard, & seasonings.

6.Pour on potato mixture & Top with the cheese.

7.Bake for 10-12 minutes until eggs are set.

8.Broil for 1-2 min.

9.Remove from oven & cool 5 min before cutting.

10Serve warm and enjoy.

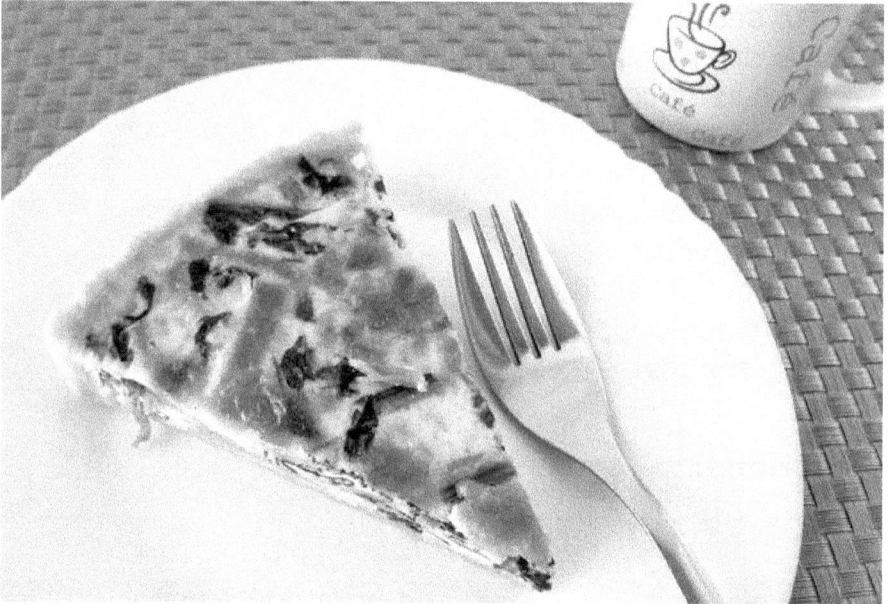

Creamy parsley soutte

Preparation time: 5 minutes
Cooking time: 5 minutes
Servings: 4

Ingredients:

25 g flour
25 g butter
1 handful parsley
Salt to taste
1 cup milk pepper (to taste)

Directions:

1.take saucepan & melt butter on moderate heat.

2.Stir in flour & mustard.

3.Stir thoroughly & form a thick paste.

4.Cook gently for 2-3 minutes.

5.Gradually whisk in milk.

6.Bring a boil, lower heat, & simmer 5 min,

7.The sauce should be quite & thick.

8.If too thick, then add a little more milk to have a smooth consistency.

9.Add parsley & stir well.

10.Season with a pinch of salt & black pepper grinds.

11. Taste & add more if needed.

12. Keep sauce warm.

13. Serve & enjoy.

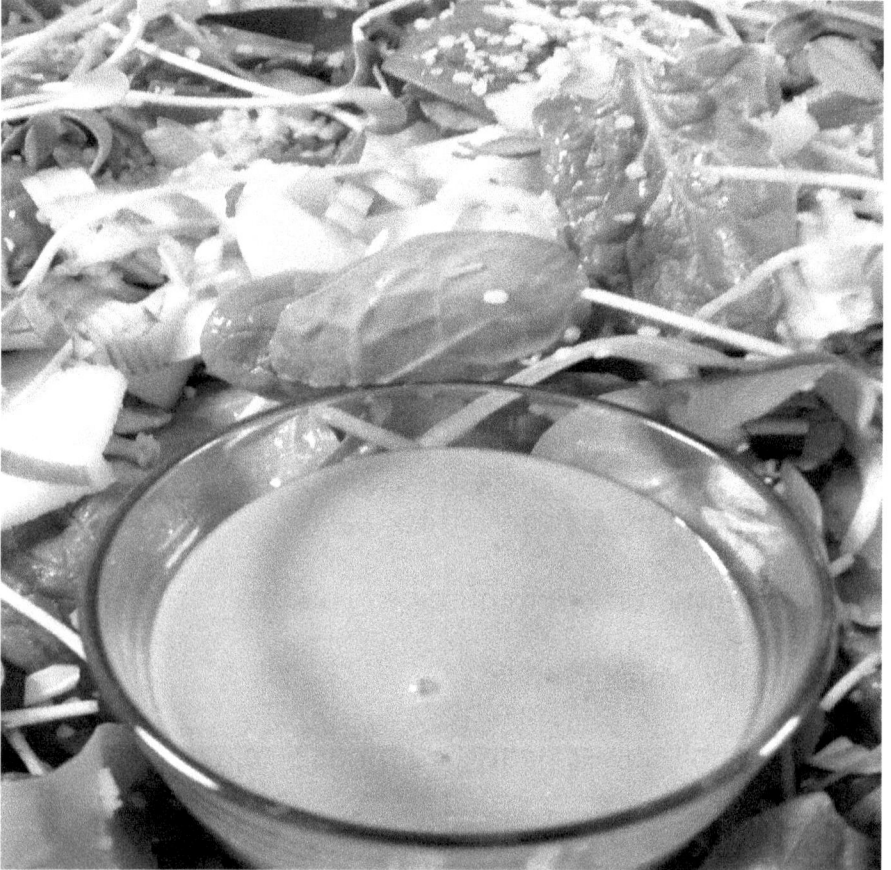

Tofu with Cauliflower

Preparation Time: 5 minutes
Cooking Time: 45 minutes
Servings: 2

Ingredients:

¼ cup red pepper, seeded
1 Thai chili, cut in two halves, seeded cloves of garlic
1 tsp of olive oil
1 pinch of cumin
1 pinch of coriander Juice of a half lemon
8oz tofu
8oz cauliflower, roughly chopped
1 ½oz. red onions, chopped
1 tsp finely chopped ginger
1 teaspoons turmeric
1oz dried tomatoes, finely chopped
1oz parsley, chopped

Directions:

1.Preheat oven to 400 °F. Slice the peppers and put them in an ovenproof dish with chili and garlic.

2.Pour some olive oil over it, add the dried herbs and put it in the oven until the peppers are soft about 20 minutes).

3.Let it cool down, put the peppers together with the lemon juice in a blender and work it into a soft mass.

4.Cut the tofu in half and divide the halves into triangles.

5.Place the tofu in a small casserole dish, cover with the paprika mixture and place in the oven for about 20 minutes.

6.Chop the cauliflower until the pieces are smaller than a grain of rice.

7.Then, in a small saucepan, heat the garlic, onions, chili and gingervwith olive oil until they become transparent. Add turmeric and cauliflower mix well and heat again.

8.Remove from heat and add parsley and tomatoes mix well. Serve with the tofu in the sauce.

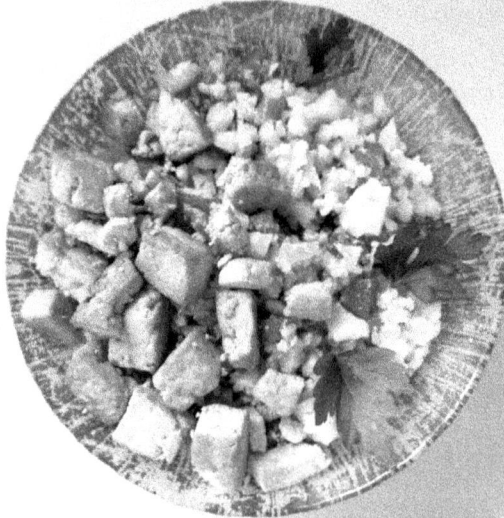

Sweet and Sour Pan

Preparation Time: 30 minutes
Cooking Time: 0 minutes
Servings: 2

Ingredients:
1 tbsp. Coconut oil pieces
Red onion pieces yellow bell pepper
12oz White cabbage
6oz Pak choi
1 ½oz. Mung bean sprouts
Pineapple slices
1 ½oz. Cashew nuts
¼ cup Apple cider vinegar tbsp.
Coconut blossom sugar 11/2 tbsp.
Tomato paste
1 tsp Coconut-Aminos
1 tsp Arrowroot powder
¼ cup Water

Directions:

1.Roughly cut the vegetables. Mix the arrow root with five tbsp. of cold water into a paste.

2.Then put all the other ingredients for the sauce in a saucepan and add the arrowroot paste for binding.

3.Melt the coconut oil in a pan and fry the onion. Add the bell pepper, cabbage, pak choi and bean sprouts and stir-fry until the vegetables become a little softer.

4.Add the pineapple and cashew nuts and stir a few more times. Pour a little sauce over the wok dish and serve.

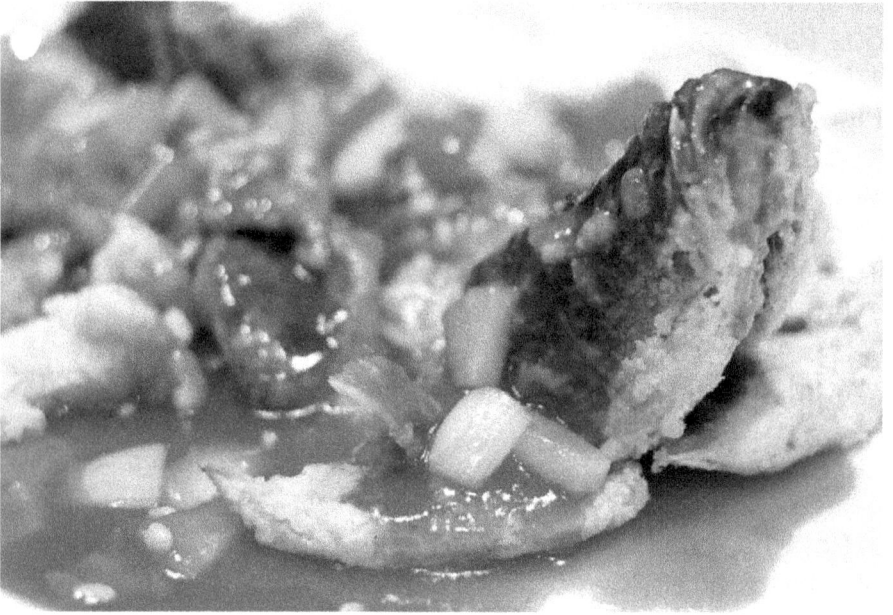

Goat's Cheese and Tomato Pizza

Preparation Time: 5 minutes
Cooking Time: 50 minutes
Servings: 2

Ingredients:

8oz buckwheat flour teaspoons dried yeast
Pinch of salt
5fl oz. slightly water
1 teaspoon olive oil
For the Topping:
oz. feta cheese, crumbled
3oz passata or tomato paste
1 tomato, sliced
1 red onion, finely chopped
1 oz. rocket arugula leaves, chopped

Directions:

1.In a bowl, combine all the ingredients for the pizza
dough and stand for at least an hour until it has
doubled in size. Roll the dough out to a size to suit you.

2.Spoon the passata onto the base and add the rest of
the toppings.

3.Bake in the oven at 200C/400F for 15-20 minutes or
until browned at the edges and crispy and serve.

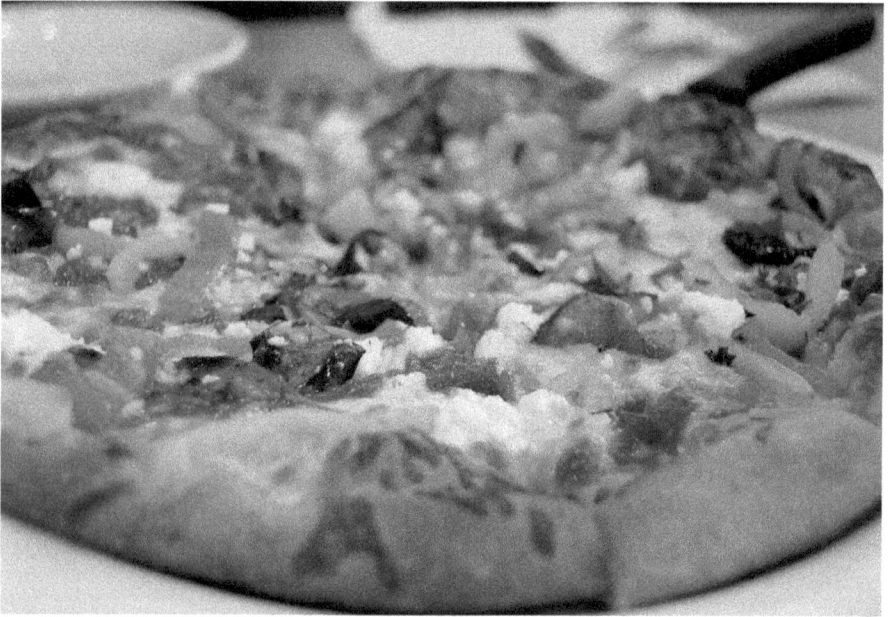

Buckwheat with Onions

Preparation Time: 10 minutes
Cooking Time: 40 minutes
Servings: 4

Ingredients:
1 cups of buckwheat, rinsed medium red onions,
chopped 1 big white onion, chopped
oz. extra-virgin olive oil cups of water
Salt and pepper, to taste

Directions:

1.Soak the buckwheat in the warm water for around 10 minutes. Then add in the buckwheat to your pot. Add in the water, salt and pepper to your pot and stir well.

2.Close the lid and cook for about 30-35 minutes until the buckwheat is ready. In the meantime, in a skillet, heat the extra-virgin olive oil and fry the chopped onions for 15 minutes until clear and caramelized.

3.Add some salt and pepper and mix well. Portion the buckwheat into four bowls or mugs. Then dollop each bowl with the onions. Remember that this dish should be served warm.

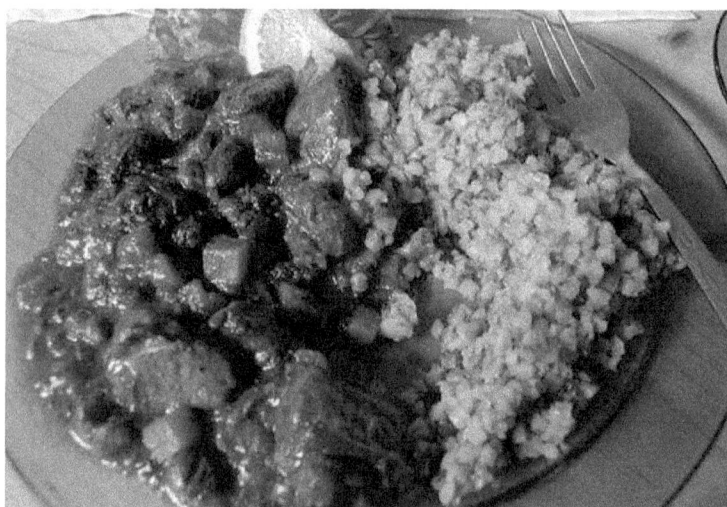

Miso Caramelized Tofu

Preparation Time: 55 minutes
Cooking Time: 15 minutes
Servings: 2

Ingredients:

1 tbsp. mirin
¾ oz. miso paste
¼ oz. firm tofu
1 ½ oz. celery, trimmed
1 ¼ oz. red onion
¼ oz. zucchini
1 bird's eye chili
1 garlic clove, finely chopped
1 tsp. fresh ginger, finely chopped
1 ⅝ oz. kale, chopped
1 tsp. sesame seeds
1 ¼ oz. buckwheat
1 tsp. ground turmeric
1 tsp. extra virgin olive oil
1 tsp. tamari (or soy sauce)

Directions:

1.Pre-heat your over to 400°F. Cover a tray with parchment paper. Combine the mirin and miso. Dice the tofu and let it marinate it in the mirin-miso mixture. Chop the vegetables (except for the kale) at a diagonal angle to produce long slices.

2.Using a steamer, cook for the kale for 5 minutes and set aside. Disperse the tofu across the lined tray and garnish with sesame seeds.

3.Roast for 20 minutes, or until caramelized. Rinse the buckwheat using running water and a sieve.

4.Add to a pan of boiling water alongside turmeric and cook the buckwheat according to the packet instructions.

5.Heat the oil in a skillet over high heat. Toss in the vegetables, herbs and spices then fry for 2-3 minutes. Reduce to a medium heat and fry for a further 5 minutes or until cooked but still crunchy.

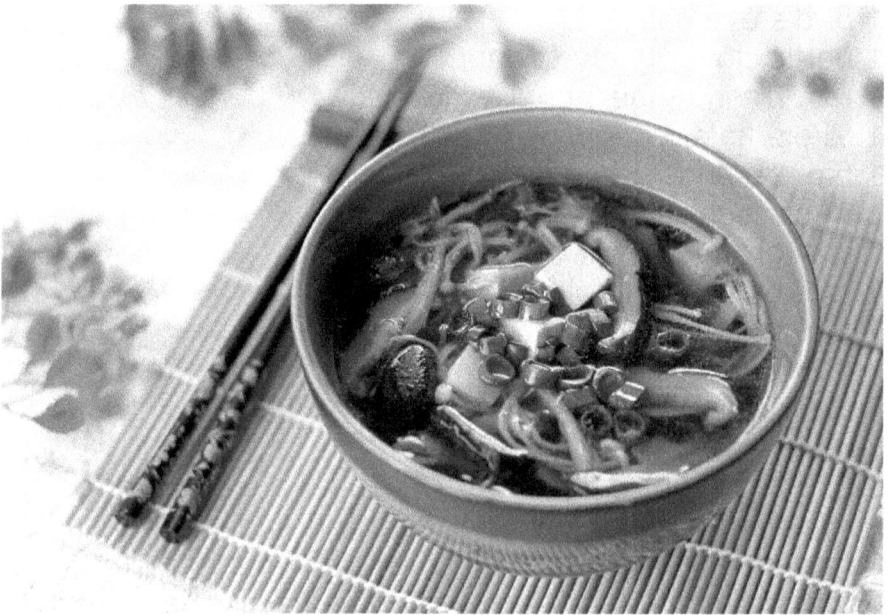

Halibut with Garlic Spinach

Preparation Time: 10 minutes
Cooking Time: 7 minutes
Servings: 2

Ingredients:

(4-ounce) halibut fillets,
1 inch thick
½ lemon (about one teaspoon juice)
1 teaspoon salt,
¼ teaspoon freshly ground black pepper (divided)
½ teaspoon cayenne pepper
1 teaspoon olive oil
cloves garlic
½ cup chopped red onion
cups fresh baby spinach leaves

Directions:

1.Preheat the broiler and place an oven rack 4 to 5 inches below the heat source. Line a baking sheet with aluminum foil.

2.Squeeze the lemon half over the fish fillets, then season each side with ½ teaspoon of the salt, pepper, and cayenne. Place the fish on the pan and broil for 7 to 8 minutes. Turn over the fish and cook for 6 to 7 minutes more, or until flaky.

3.Meanwhile, heat the olive oil in a small skillet over medium heat. Add the garlic and onion, and sauté for 2 minutes. Add the spinach and remaining ½ teaspoon salt, and sauté for 2 minutes more. Remove from the heat and cover to keep warm.

4.To serve, divide the spinach between two plates and top each portion with a fish fillet. Serve hot.

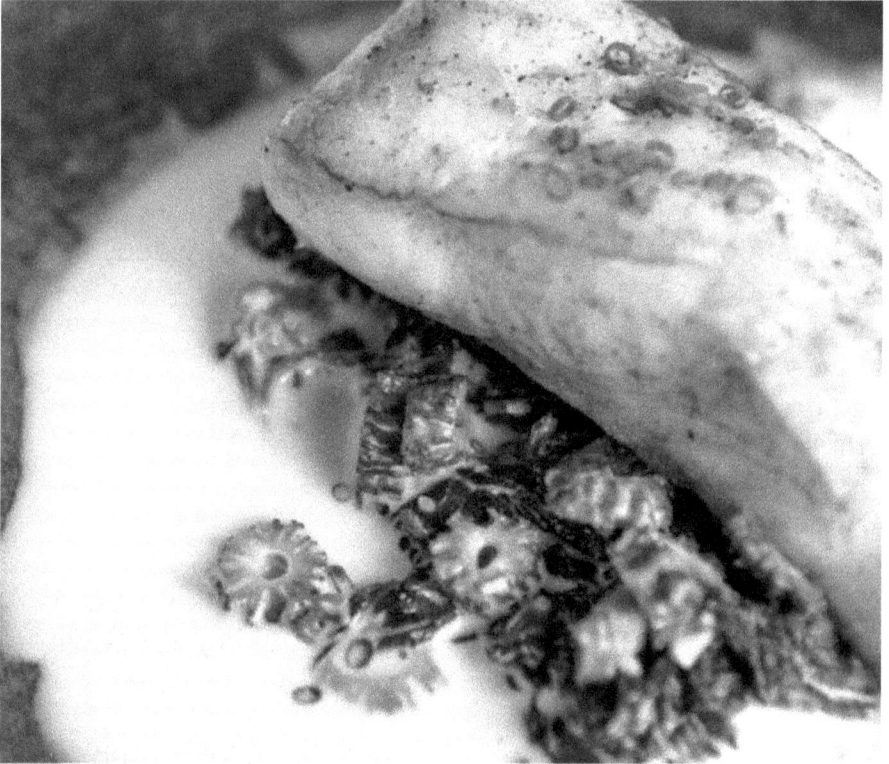

Quinoa Pilaf

Preparation Time: 30 minutes
Cooking Time: 20 minutes
Servings: 4

Ingredients:

tablespoons extra virgin olive oil
1/2 medium yellow onion, finely chopped
1/4 bell pepper, finely chopped
1 garlic clove, minced tablespoons pine nuts
1 cup uncooked quinoa cups of water
Pinch freshly ground black pepper
tablespoons chopped fresh mint
tablespoons chopped fresh basil or Thai basil*
1 tablespoon chopped fresh chives (or green onions including the greens)
1 small cucumber, peeled, seeds removed, chopped
Salt and pepper

Directions:

1.If you recommend washing it, check your quinoa box, place the quinoa in a large sieve, and rinse it to remove water. (Some brands do not require washing).

2.Onions, Peppers, garlic, pine nuts: Heat 1 tbsp. put the olive oil over medium-high heat in a pot of 1/1 to 2 quarts.

3.Add and cook onions, rusty peppers, garlic and pine nuts, occasionally stirring until the onions are translucent but not browned.

4.Add quinoa: add and cook uncooked quinoa, occasionally stirring for a few minutes. You can toast a little quinoa for some bread.

5.Add water, salt, stir: Add two glasses of water and a teaspoon of salt. Bring to a boil and reduce heat so that cheese and water shine while the pot is partially covered (enough for steam).

6.Cook for 20 minutes or until quinoa is thin and liquid is absorbed. Remove from heat and serve in a large bowl.

7.Fill with a fork. Add olive oil, mint, basil, onion, and cucumber: add over low heat and add another tablespoon of olive oil. In chopped mint, mix basil, onion and cucumber.

8.Add salt and pepper to taste. Chill or cool at room temperature.

Crispy Chickpeas with Green Beans

Preparation Time: 30 minutes
Cooking Time: 10 minutes
Servings: 4

Ingredients:

1 can chickpeas, rinsed
1 tsp. whole coriander
1 lb. green beans, trimmed
1 tbsp. olive oil, divided
Kosher salt and freshly ground black pepper
1 tsp. cumin seeds
Grilled lemons, for serving

Directions:

1.Heat grill to medium. Gather chickpeas, coriander, cumin, and 1 tbsp. oil in a medium cast-iron skillet. Put skillet on grill and cook chickpeas, mixing occasionally, until golden brown and coriander begins to pop, 5 to 6 minutes. Season with salt and pepper.

2.Transfer to a bowl. Add green beans and remaining tbsp. olive oil to the skillet. Add salt and pepper. Cook, turning once, until charred and barely tender, 3 to 4 minutes.

3.Toss green beans with chickpea mixture and serve with grilled lemons alongside.

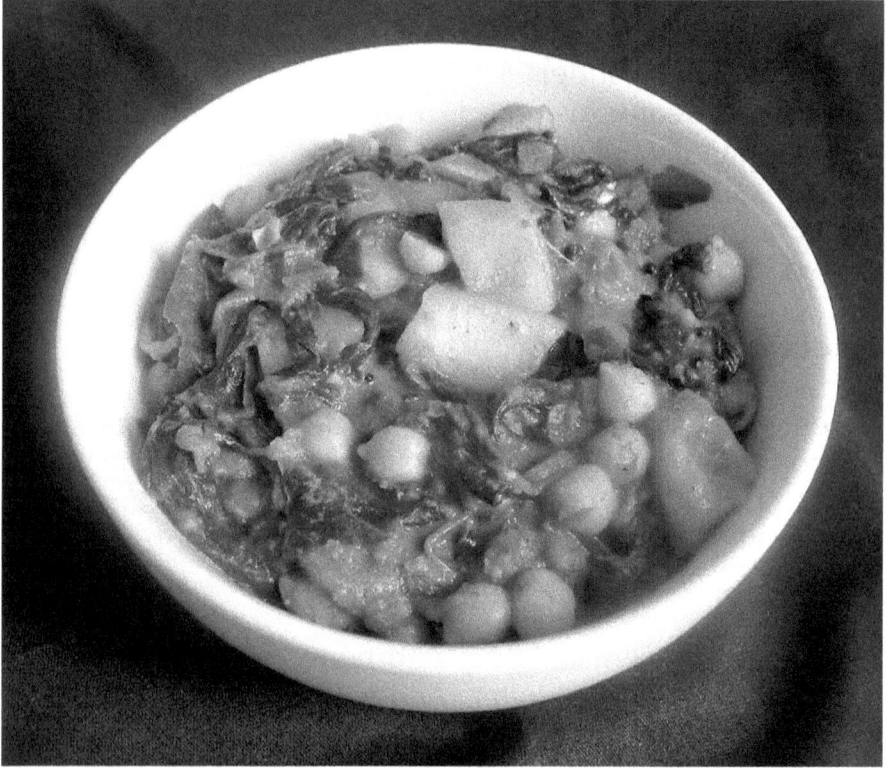

Turkey Satay Skewers

Preparation Time: 15 minutes
Cooking Time: 20 minutes
Servings: 4

Ingredients:

250g (9oz) turkey breast, cubed
25g (1oz) smooth peanut butter
1 clove of garlic, crushed
½ small bird's eye chilli (or more if you like it hotter),
finely chopped
½ teaspoon ground turmeric
200mls (7fl oz.) coconut milk
1 teaspoons soy sauce

Directions:

1.Combine the coconut milk, peanut butter, turmeric,
soy sauce, garlic and chilli.

2.Add the turkey pieces to the bowl and stir them until
they are completely coated. Push the turkey onto metal
skewers.

3.Place the satay skewers on a barbeque or under a hot
grill (broiler) and cook for 4-5 minutes on each side,
until they are completely cooked.

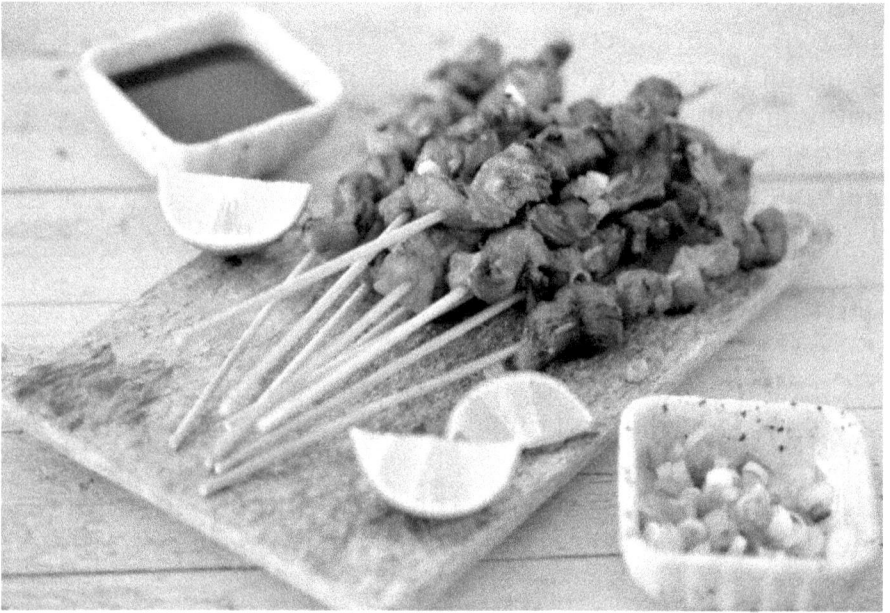

Salmon & Capers

Preparation Time: 15 minutes
Cooking Time: 20 minutes
Servings: 2

Ingredients:

75g (3oz) Greek yogurt salmon fillets, skin removed
1teaspoons Dijon Mustard
1 tablespoon capers, chopped teaspoons fresh parsley
Zest of 1 lemon

Directions:

1.In a bowl, mix the yogurt, mustard, lemon zest, parsley and capers. Thoroughly coat the salmon in the mixture.

2 Place the salmon under a hot grill (broiler) and cook for 3-4 minutes on each side, or until the fish is cooked.

3 Serve with mashed potatoes and vegetables or a large green leafy salad.

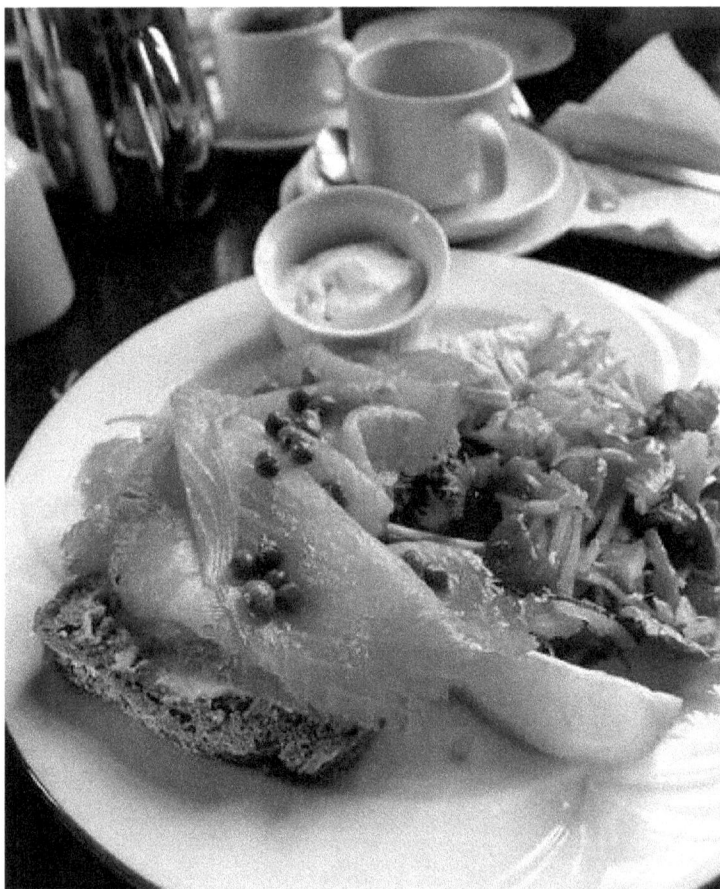

Prawn & Coconut Curry

Preparation Time: 10 minutes
Cooking Time: 25 minutes
Servings: 4

Ingredients:

400g (14oz) tinned chopped tomatoes
400g (14oz) large prawns (shrimps), shelled and raw
25g (1oz) fresh coriander (cilantro) chopped
1 red onions, finely chopped
1 cloves of garlic, crushed bird's eye chillies
½ teaspoon ground coriander (cilantro)
½ teaspoon turmeric
400mls (14fl oz.) coconut milk
1 tablespoons olive oil
Juice of 1 lime

Directions:

1.Place the onions, garlic, tomatoes, chillies, lime juice, turmeric, ground coriander (cilantro), chillies and half of the fresh coriander (cilantro) blender and blitz until you have a smooth curry paste.

2.Heat the olive oil in a frying pan, add the paste and cook for 2 minutes. Stir in the coconut milk and warm it thoroughly.

3.Add the prawns (shrimps) to the paste and cook them until they have turned pink and are completely cooked. Stir in the fresh coriander (cilantro). Serve with rice.

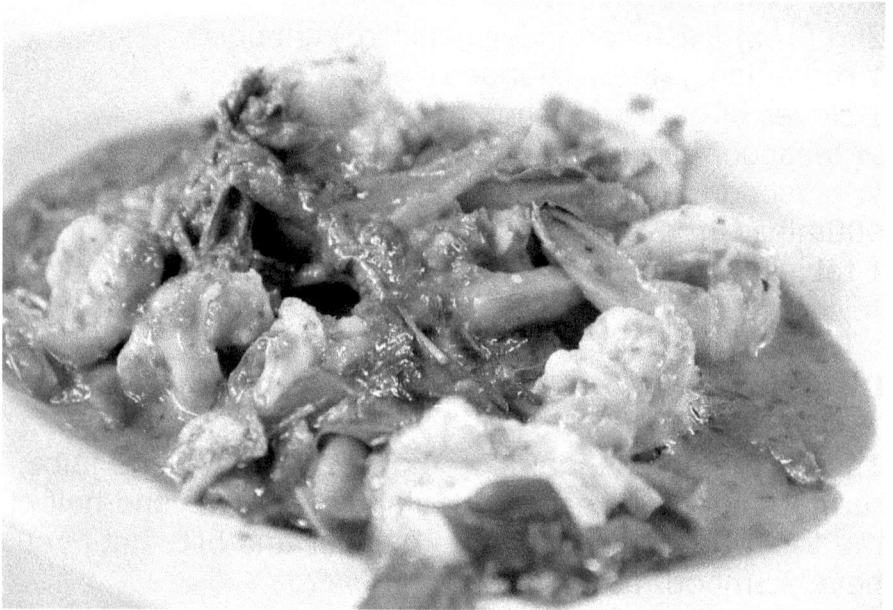

Kale White Bean Pork Soup

Preparation Time: 5 minutes
Cooking Time: 45 minutes
Servings: 4-6

Ingredients:
1 tbsp. extra-virgin olive oil
1 tbsp. chili powder
1 tbsp. jalapeno hot sauce pounds bone-in pork chops
Salt
1 stalks celery, chopped
1 large white onion, chopped cloves
1 garlic, chopped
3 cups chicken broth cups diced tomatoes
2 cups cooked white beans cups packed kale

Directions:

1.Preheat the broiler.

2.Whisk hot sauce, 1 tbsp. olive oil and chili powder in a bowl.

3.Season the pork chops with ½ tsp salt.

4.Rub chops with the spice mixture on both sides and place them on a rack set over a baking sheet.

5.Set aside.

6.Heat 1 tbsp. olive oil in a pot over medium heat.

7.Add the celery, garlic, onion, and the remaining 2 tbsp. chili powder.

8.Cook until onions are translucent, stirring (approx. 8 minutes).

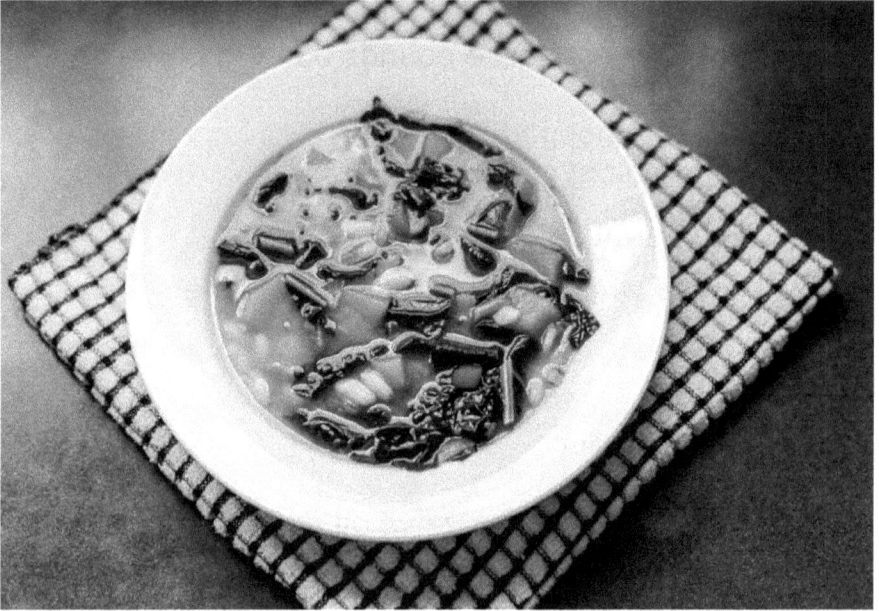

Salad

Preparation Time: 5 minutes
Cooking Time: 40 minutes
Servings: 3

Ingredients:

100g red chicory
150g tuna flakes in brine, drained
100g cucumber
25g rocket
1 cups kalamata olives, pitted
Hard-boiled eggs, peeled and quartered tomatoes, chopped
1 tbsp. fresh parsley, chopped 1 red onion, chopped
1 celery stalk
1 tbsp. capers
1 tbsp. garlic vinaigrette

Directions:

1.Combine all ingredients in a bowl and serve.

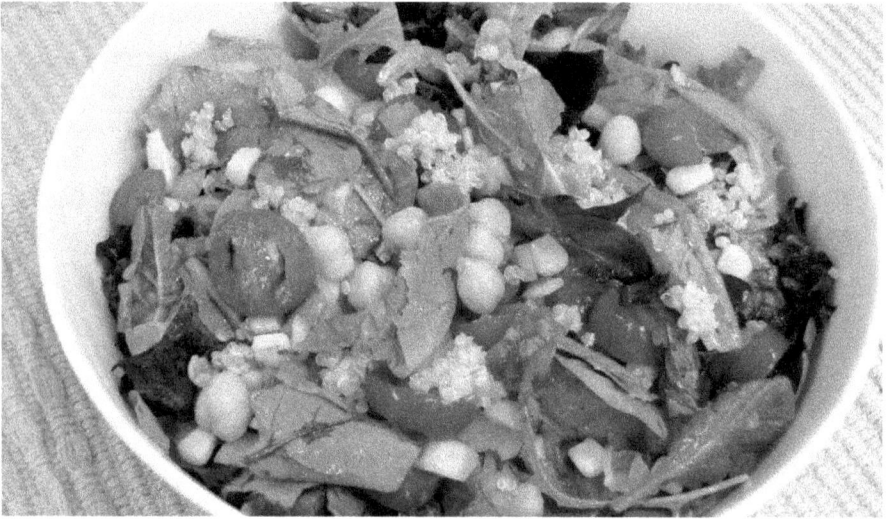

Turkey Curry

Preparation Time: 5 minutes
Cooking Time: 40 minutes
Servings: 3

Ingredients:

450g (1lb), turkey breasts, chopped
100g (3½ oz.) fresh rocket (arugula) leaves
1 cloves garlic, chopped
1 tsp medium curry powder
1 tsp turmeric powder
1 tbsp. fresh coriander (cilantro), finely chopped bird's
eye chilies, chopped
1 red onions, chopped
400ml (14fl oz.) full-fat coconut milk
1.tbsp. olive oil

Directions:

1.Heat the olive oil in a saucepan, add the chopped red
onions and cook them for around 5 minutes or until
soft.

2.Stir in the garlic and the turkey and cook it for 7-8
minutes.

3.Stir in the turmeric, chilies and curry powder then add
the coconut milk and coriander cilantro).

4.Bring it to the boil, reduce the heat and simmer for
around 10 minutes. Scatter the rocket (arugula) onto
plates and spoon the curry on top.

5.Serve alongside brown rice.

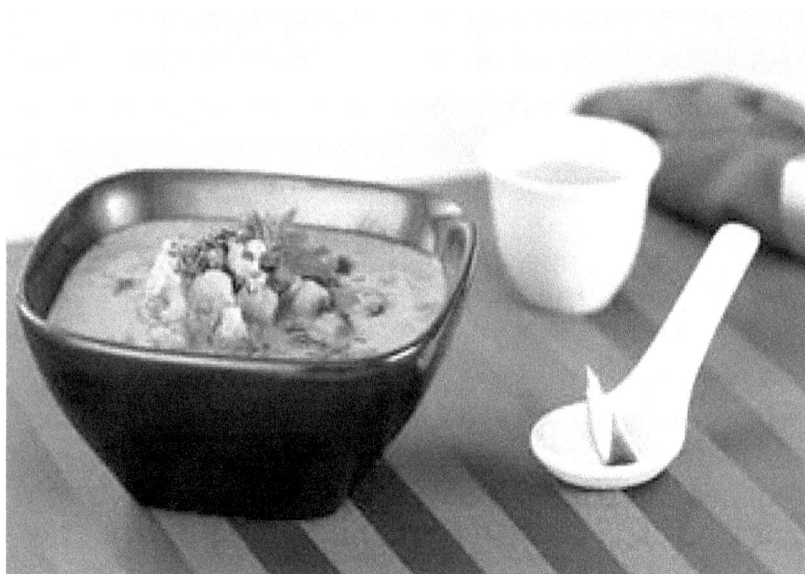

Tofu and Curry

Preparation Time: 5 minutes
Cooking Time: 36 minutes
Servings: 4

Ingredients:

oz. dried lentils (red preferably)
1 cup boiling water
1 cup frozen edamame (soy) beans
oz. (½ of most packages) firm tofu, chopped into cubes
tomatoes, chopped
1 lime juices
5-6 kale leaves, stalks removed and torn
1 large onion, chopped
1 cloves garlic, peeled and grated
1 large chunk of ginger, grated
½ red chili pepper, deseeded (use less if too much)
½ tsp ground turmeric
¼ tsp cayenne pepper
1 tsp paprika
½ tsp ground cumin
1 tsp salt
1 tbsp. olive oil

Directions:

1.Add the onion, sauté in the oil for few minutes then add the chili, garlic, and ginger for a bit longer until wilted but not burned.

2.Add the seasonings, then the lentils and stir

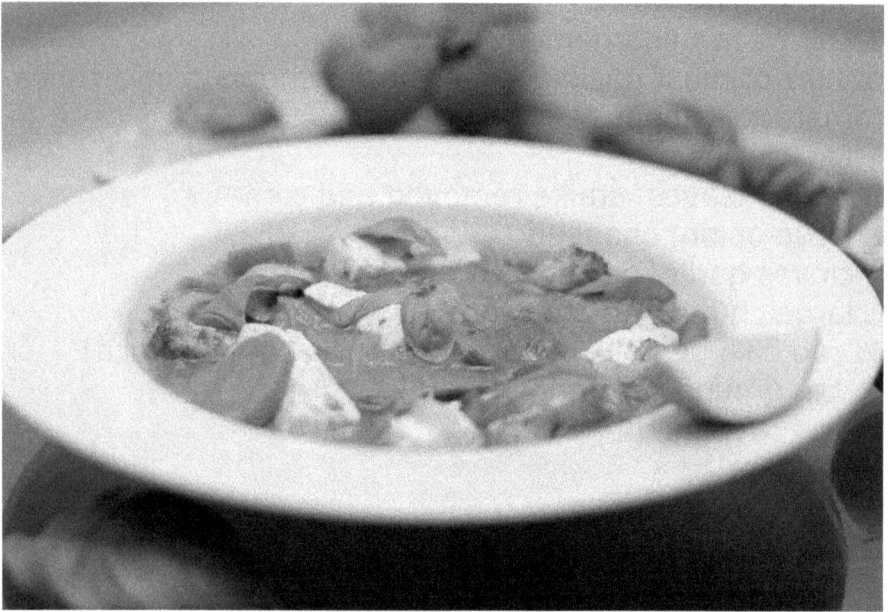

Chicken and Bean Casserole

Preparation Time: 5 minutes
Cooking Time: 40 minutes
Servings: 3

Ingredients:

400g (14oz) chopped tomatoes
400g (14oz) tinned cannellini beans or haricot beans
Chicken thighs, skin removed
3 carrots, peeled and finely chopped
1 red onions, chopped
sticks of celery large mushrooms
2 red peppers (bell peppers), de-seeded and chopped
1 clove of garlic
1 tbsp. soy sauce
1 tbsp. olive oil
liters (3 pints) chicken stock (broth)

Directions:

1.Heat the olive oil in a saucepan, add the garlic and onions and cook for 5 minutes.

2.Add in the chicken and cook for 5 minutes then add the carrots, cannellini beans, celery, red peppers (bell peppers) and mushrooms.

3.Pour in the stock (broth) soy sauce and tomatoes.

4.Bring it to the boil, reduce the heat and simmer for 45 minutes.

5.Serve with rice or new potatoes.

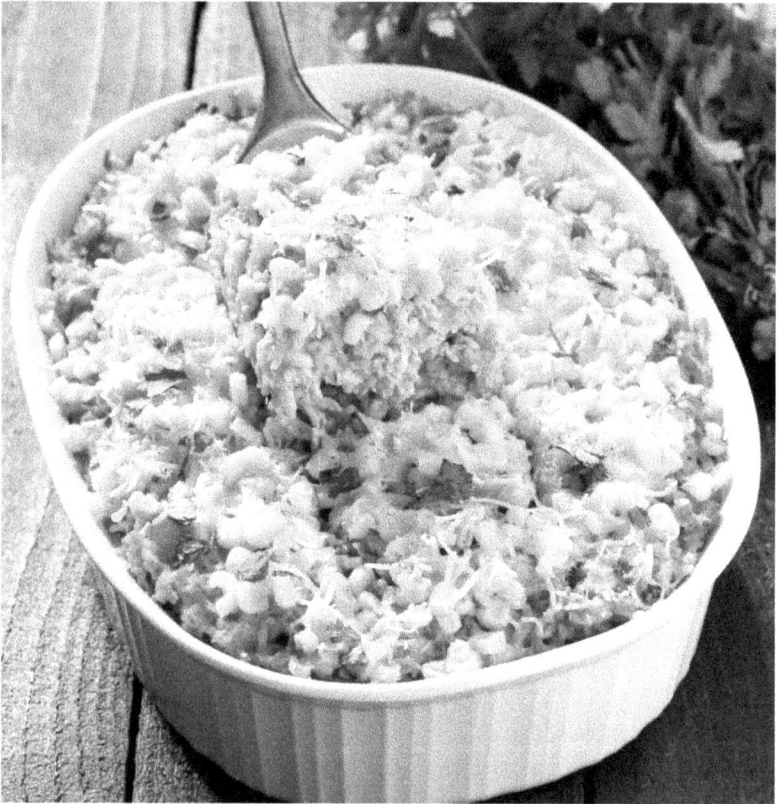

Prawn and Coconut Curry

Preparation Time: 5 minutes
Cooking Time: 35 minutes
Servings: 3

Ingredients:

400g (14oz) tinned chopped tomatoes
400g (14oz) large prawns (shrimps), shelled and raw
25g (1oz) fresh coriander (cilantro) chopped
1 red onions, finely chopped
1 cloves of garlic, crushed bird's eye chilies
½ tsp ground coriander (cilantro)
½ tsp turmeric
400ml (14fl oz.) coconut milk
1 tbsp. olive oil
Juice of 1 lime

Directions:

1.Place the onions, garlic, tomatoes, chilies, lime juice, turmeric, ground coriander (cilantro), chilies and half of the fresh coriander (cilantro) into a blender and blitz until you have a smooth curry paste.

2.Heat the olive oil in a frying pan, add the paste and cook for 2 minutes.

3.Stir in the coconut milk and warm it thoroughly.

4.Add the prawns (shrimps) to the paste and cook them until they have turned pink and are thoroughly cooked.

5.Stir in the fresh coriander (cilantro).

6.Serve with rice.

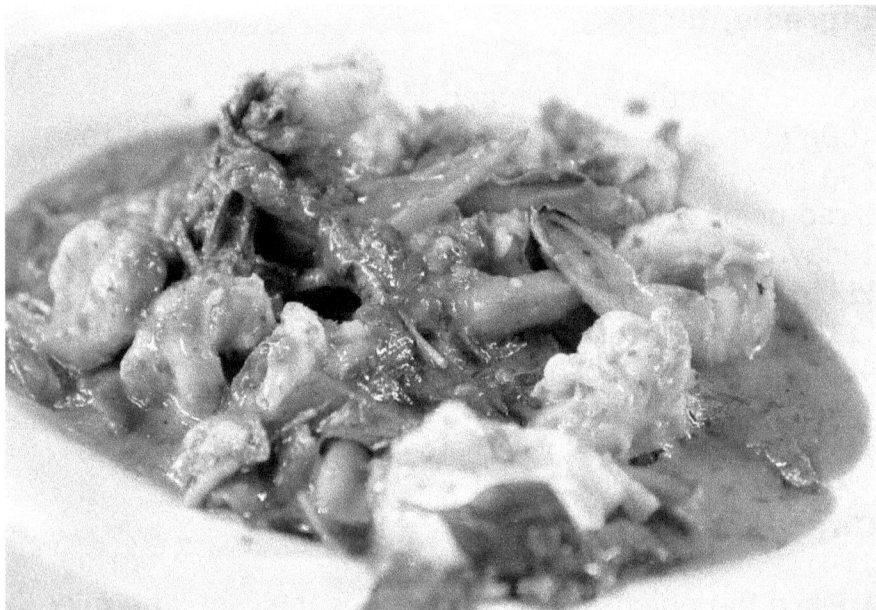

Moroccan Chicken Casserole

Preparation Time: 5 minutes
Cooking Time: 20 minutes
Servings: 3

Ingredients:

250g (9oz) tinned chickpeas (garbanzo beans) drained
500g chicken breasts, cubed
Medjool dates halved dried apricots, halved
1 red onion, sliced
1 carrot, chopped
1 tsp ground cumin
1 tsp cinnamon
1 tsp ground turmeric
1 bird's eye chili, chopped
600ml (1 pint) chicken stock (broth)
25g (1oz) corn flour
60ml (2fl oz.) water tbsp. fresh coriander

Directions:

1.Place the chicken, chickpeas (garbanzo beans), onion, carrot, chili, cumin, turmeric, cinnamon, and stock (broth) into a large saucepan.

2.Bring it to the boil, reduce the heat and simmer for 25 minutes.

3.Add in the dates and apricots and simmer for 10 minutes.

4.In a cup, mix the corn flour with the water until it becomes a smooth paste.

5.Pour the mixture into the saucepan and stir until it thickens.

6.Add in the coriander (cilantro) and mix well.

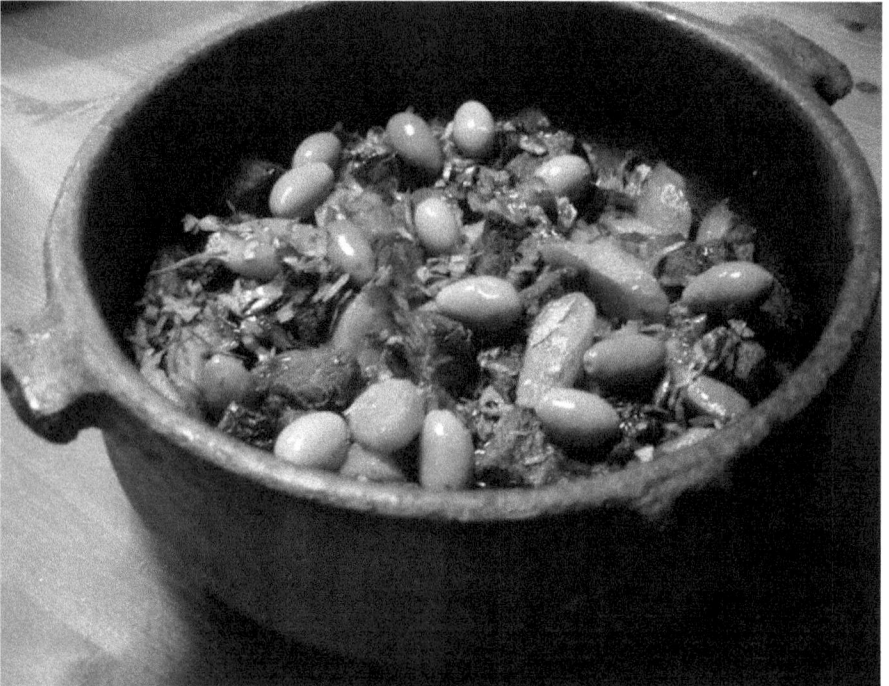

Chili con Carne

Preparation Time: 5 minutes
Cooking Time: 30 minutes
Servings: 3

Ingredients:

450g (1lb) lean minced beef
400g (14oz) chopped tomatoes
200g (7oz) red kidney beans
1 tbsp. tomato purée
1 cloves of garlic, crushed red onions, chopped
bird's eye chilies, finely chopped
1 red pepper (bell pepper), chopped
1 stick of celery, finely chopped
1 tbsp. cumin
1 tbsp. turmeric
1 tbsp. cocoa powder
400ml (14 oz.) beef stock (broth)
175ml (6fl oz.) red wine
1 tbsp. olive oil

Directions:

1.Heat the oil in a large saucepan, add the onion and cook for 5 minutes.

2.Add in the garlic, celery, chili, turmeric, and cumin and cook for 2 minutes before adding then meat then cook for another 5 minutes.

3.Pour in the stock (broth), red wine, tomatoes, tomato purée, red pepper (bell pepper), kidney beans and cocoa powder.

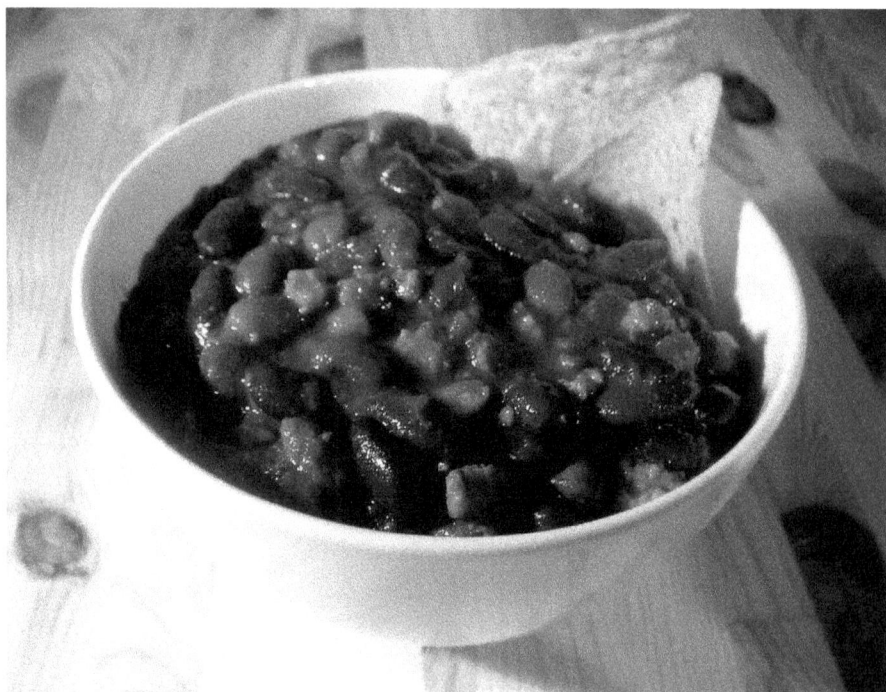

Tofu Thai Curry

Preparation Time: 5 minutes
Cooking Time: 30 minutes
Servings: 3

Ingredients:

400g (14oz) tofu, diced
200g (7oz) sugar snap peas
5cm (2-inch) chunk fresh ginger root, peeled and finely chopped
1 red onions, chopped
1 cloves of garlic, crushed bird's eye chilies
1 tbsp. tomato puree
1 stalk of lemongrass, inner stalks only
1 tbsp. fresh coriander (cilantro), chopped
1 tsp cumin
300ml (½ pint) coconut milk
200ml (7fl oz.) vegetable stock (broth)
1 tbsp. virgin olive oil
juice of 1 lime

Directions:

1.Heat the oil in a frying pan, add the onion and cook for 4 minutes.

2.Add in the chilies, cumin, ginger, and garlic and cook for 2 minutes.

3.Add the tomato puree, lemongrass, sugar-snap peas, lime juice and tofu and cook for 2 minutes.

4.Pour in the stock (broth), coconut milk and coriander (cilantro) and simmer for 5 minutes.

5.Serve with brown rice or buckwheat and a handful of rockets (arugula) leaves on the side.

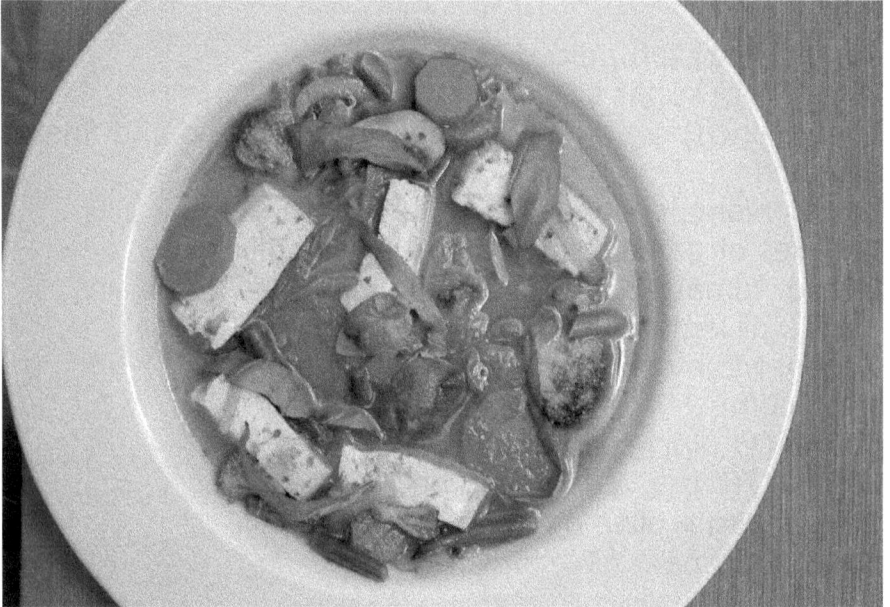

Roasted Artichoke Hearts

Preparation Time: 5 minutes
Cooking Time: 40 minutes
Servings: 3

Ingredients:
1 cans artichoke hearts
1 garlic cloves, quartered
1tsp extra virgin olive oil
1 tsp dried oregano
Salt and pepper, to taste
2-3 tbsp. lemon juice, to serve

Directions:

1.Preheat oven to 375F.

2.Drain the artichoke hearts and rinse them very thoroughly.

3.Toss them in garlic, oregano, and olive oil.

4.Arrange the artichoke hearts in a baking dish and bake for about 45 minutes tossing a few times if desired.

5.Season with salt and pepper and serve with lemon juice.

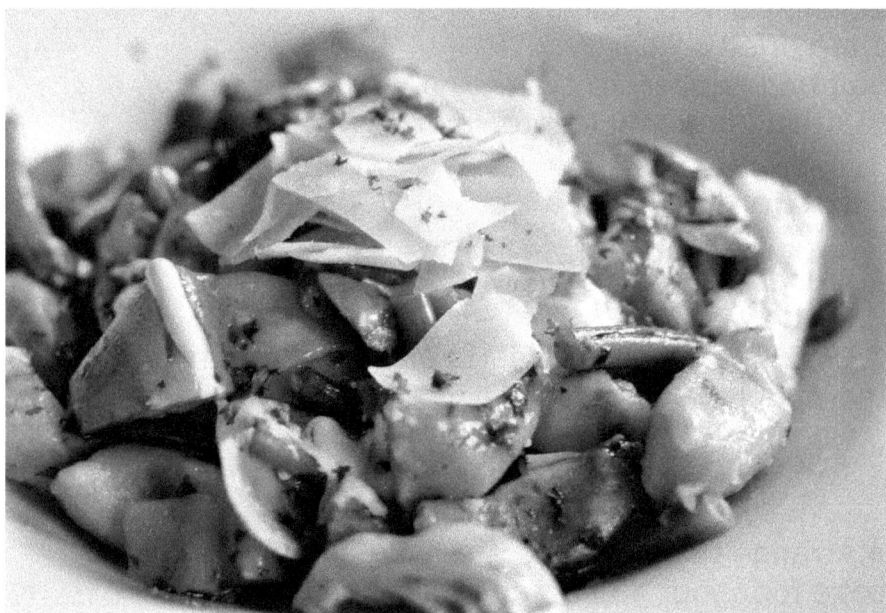

Beef Broth

Preparation Time: 5 minutes
Cooking Time: 40 minutes
Servings: 3

Ingredients:

4-5 pounds beef bones and few veal bones
1 pound of stew meat (chuck or flank steak) cut into 2-inch chunks
Olive oil
1-2 medium red onions, peeled and quartered
1-2 large carrots, cut into 1-2-inch segments
1 celery rib, cut into 1-inch segments
2-3 cloves of garlic, unpeeled
A handful of parsley stems and leaves
1-2 bay leaves peppercorns

Directions:

1.Heat oven to 375F.

2.Rub olive oil over the stew meat pieces, carrots, and onions.

3.Place stew meat or beef scraps, stock bones, carrots, and onions in a large roasting pan.

4.Roast in the oven for about 45 minutes, turning everything halfway through the cooking.

5.Place everything from the oven in a large stockpot.

6.Pour some boiling water in the oven pan and scrape up all the browned bits and pour all in the stockpot.

7.Add parsley, celery, garlic, bay leaves, and peppercorns to the pot.

8.Fill the pot with cold water, to 1-inch over the top of the bones.

9.Bring the stockpot to a regular simmer and then reduce the heat to low, so it just barely simmers. Cover the pot loosely and let simmer low and slow for 3-4 hours.

10.Scoop away the fat and any scum that rises to the surface occasionally.

11.After cooking, remove the bones and vegetables from the pot.

12.Strain the broth.

13.Let cool to room temperature and then put in the refrigerator.

14.The fat will solidify once the broth has chilled.

15.Discard the fat (or reuse it) and pour the broth into a jar and freeze it.

Mediterranean Pork with Olives and Rosemary

Total time - 40Minutes
Servings - 6

Ingredients:

6 Bone-in or boneless pork chops (3 4 inch thick)
¼ Dry white wine (or beef broth
2 cloves Garlic (finely chopped)
1 pinch ground cinnamon
1 tbsp Olive oil
1 Onions (large, sliced)
1 jar Ragu old world style pasta sauce
½ cup Ripe olives (sliced, pitted)

Directions:

1.Cook pork chops inside pan using 1 tablespoon of olive oil set on medium to high heat.

2.Remove pork chop from pan when it turns brown.

3.Cook onion and garlic on medium heat in the same pan, and stir periodically, until onion is done.

4.Pour wine into the pan let it boil on high heat, and prevent brown bits from attaching to the pan's bottom.

5.Return pork chop into the pan.

6.While you stir, add pasta sauce and the remaining

7.Return the lid and stir periodically for 20 minutes or until pork chop is properly cooked.

8.Decorate with fresh rosemary and extra olives. Ready to serve with hot cooked rice.

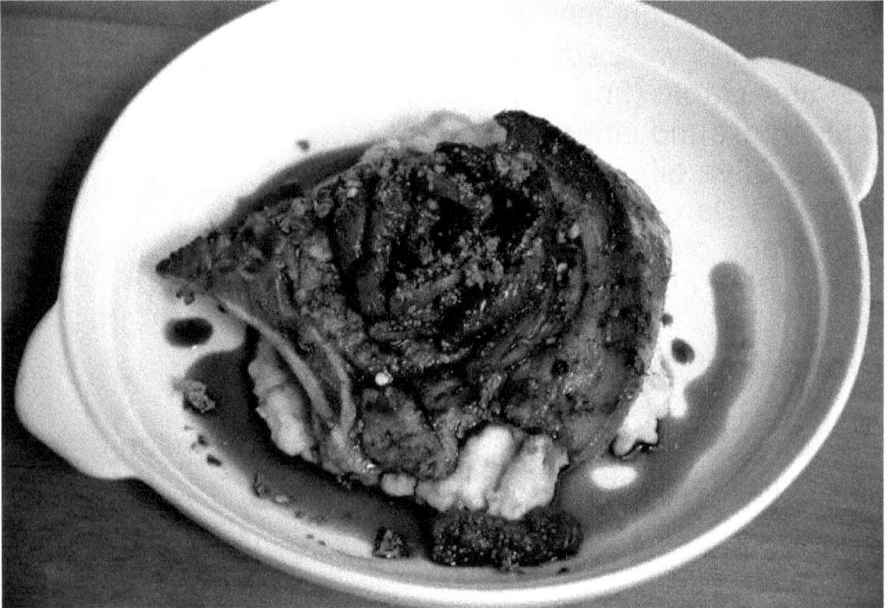

Braised Mediterranean Chicken with Rosemary Leaves

Total time – 45 Minutes
Servings - 4

Ingredients:

1tbsp Bertolli classico olive oil.
1 jar Bertolli vineyard premium collections marinara with burgundy wine sauce
2 ¾ Chicken (cut into serving pieces)
2 cloves Garlic (large, finely chopped)
¼ tsp Ground black pepper
½ cup Orange juice
1/3 cup Pitted kalamata olives (or pitted ripe olives, halved)
1 tsp Rosemary leaves (chopped, fresh, or 1 teaspoon.
2 tsp Dried rosemary leaves, crushed,optional

Directions:

1.Cook chicken inside pan using 1 tablespoon of olive oil set on medium to high heat.

2.Remove chicken from pan when it turns brown. Leave drippings in the pan.

3.Pour garlic, olives, and rosemary into the pan containing reserved drippings and cook on medium heat for 2 minutes while stirring periodically.

4.Pour orange juice, stirring and scraping up the bits that attach to the bottom of the pan.

5.Add Sauce and pepper. Continue to stir

6.Increase to high heat. Add chicken to skillet.

7.Return heat to low and close the lid. Leave to simmer for 30 minutes or until chicken is done.

8.Ready to serve with rice along with some sauce.

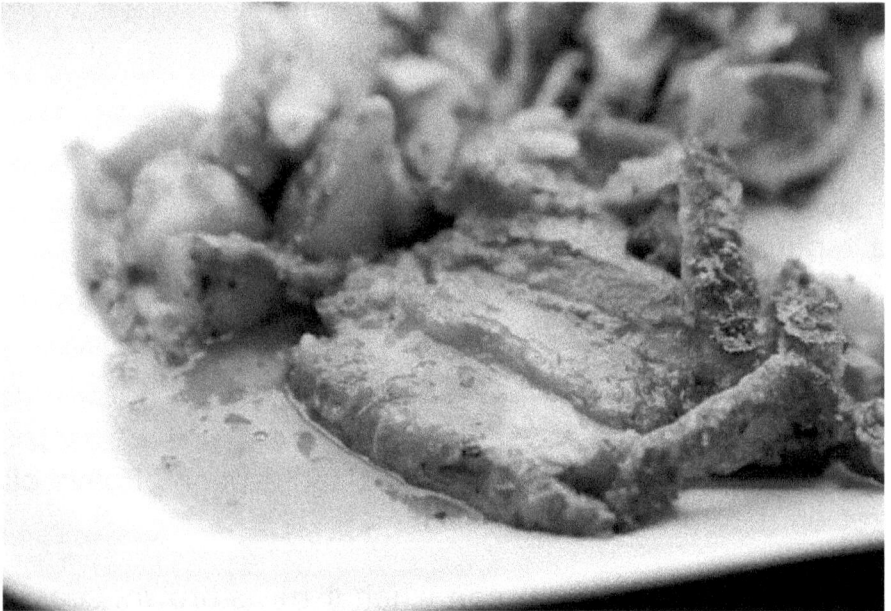

Flat Meat Pies

Preparation Time: 20 minutes
Cooking Time: 15 minutes
Servings: 4

Ingredients:

½ lb. ground beef

1 small onion, finely chopped

1 medium tomato, finely diced and strained

½ tsp. salt

½ tsp. freshly ground black pepper

2 sheets puff pastry

Directions:

1.Preheat the oven to 400°F.

2.In a medium bowl, combine the beef, onion, tomato, salt, and pepper. Set aside.

3.Line 2 baking sheets with parchment paper. Cut the puff pastry dough into 4-inch squares and lay them flat on the baking sheets.

4.Scoop about 2 tbsp. of beef mixture onto each piece of dough. Spread the meat on the dough, leaving a ½-inch edge on each side.

5.Put the meat pies in the oven and bake for 12 to 15 minutes until edges are golden brown.

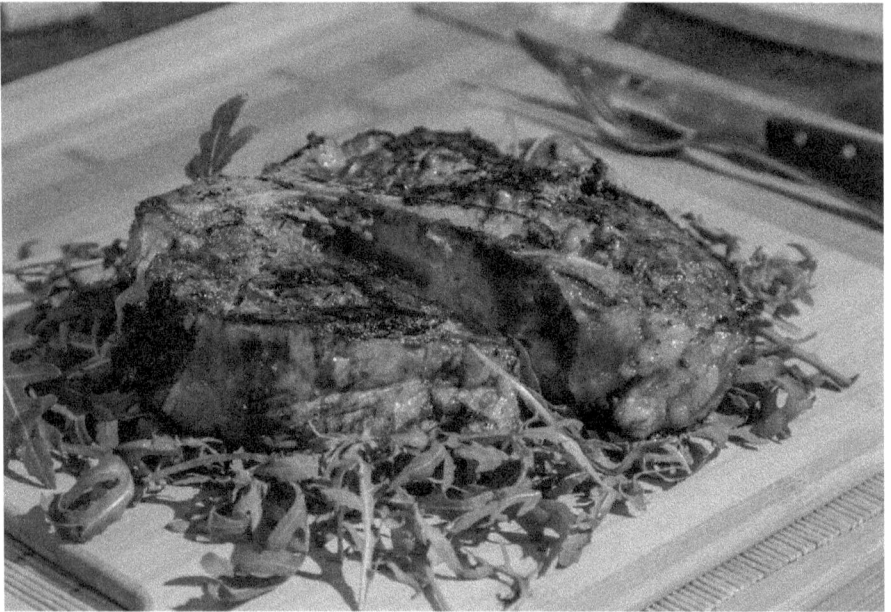

Meaty Baked Penne

Preparation Time: 10 minutes
Cooking Time: 40 minutes
Servings: 6

Ingredients:

1 lb. penne pasta
1 lb. ground beef
1 tsp. salt
1 (25-oz.) jar marinara sauce
1 (1-lb.) bag baby spinach, washed
3 cups shredded mozzarella cheese, divided

Directions:

1.Bring a large pot of salted water to a boil, add the penne, and cook for 7 minutes. Reserve 2 cups of e pasta water and drain the pasta.

2.Preheat the oven to 350°F.

3.In a large saucepan over medium heat, cook the ground beef and salt. Brown the ground beef for about 5 minutes.

4.Stir in marinara sauce, and 2 cups of pasta water. Let simmer for 5 minutes.

5.Add a handful of spinach at a time into the sauce, and cook for another 3 minutes.

6.To assemble, In a 9-by-13-inch baking dish, add the pasta and pour the pasta sauce over it. Stir in 1½ cups of the mozzarella cheese. Cover the dish with foil and bake for 20 minutes.

7.After 20 minutes, remove the foil, top with the rest of the mozzarella, and bake for another 10 minutes. Serve warm.

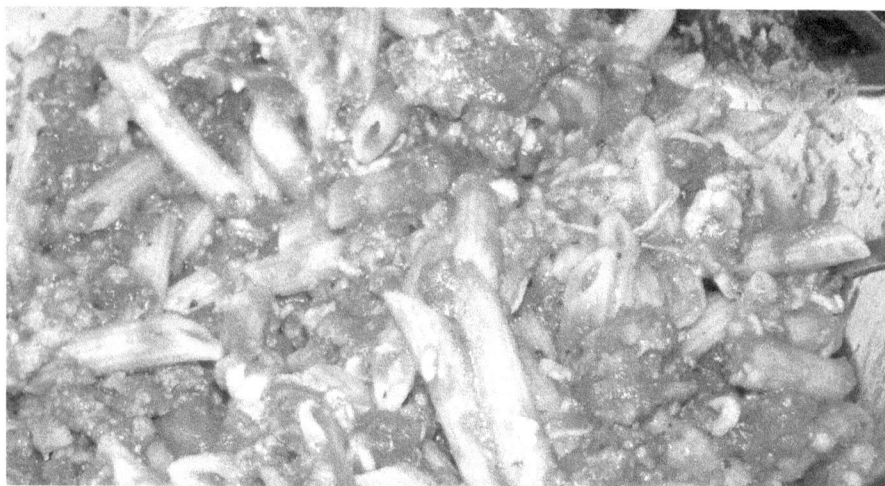

Mediterranean Pasta with Tomato Sauce and Vegetables

Preparation Time: 15 minutes
Cooking Time: 25 minutes
Servings: 8

Ingredients:

8 oz. linguine or spaghetti, cooked
1 tsp. garlic powder
1 (28 oz.) can whole peeled tomatoes, drained and sliced 1 tbsp. olive oil
1 (8 oz.) can tomato sauce
½ tsp. Italian seasoning
8 oz. mushrooms, sliced
8 oz. yellow squash, sliced
8 oz. zucchini, sliced
½ tsp. sugar
½ cup grated Parmesan cheese

Directions:

1.In a medium saucepan, mix tomato sauce, tomatoes, sugar, Italian seasoning, and garlic powder. Bring to boil on medium heat. Reduce heat to low. Cover and simmer for 20 minutes.

2.In a large skillet, heat olive oil on medium-high heat.

3.Add squash, mushrooms, and zucchini. Cook, stirring, for 4 minutes or until tender-crisp.
Stir vegetables into the tomato sauce.

4.Place pasta in a serving bowl.

5.Spoon vegetable mixture over pasta and toss to coat.

6.Top with grated Parmesan cheese.

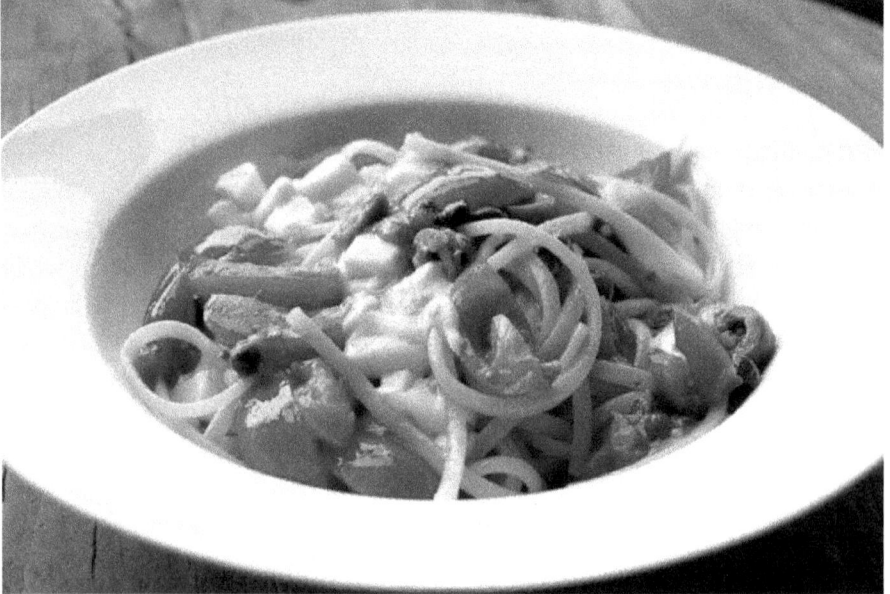

Very Vegan Patras Pasta

Preparation Time: 5 minutes
Cooking Time: 10 minutes
Servings: 6

Ingredients:

4-quarts salted water
10-oz. gluten-free and whole-grain pasta
5-cloves garlic, minced
1cup hummus
Salt and pepper
11/3-cup water
½-cup walnuts
½-cup olives
2- tbsp dried cranberries (optional)

Directions:

1.Bring the salted water to a boil for cooking the pasta.

2.In the meantime, prepare for the hummus sauce. Combine the garlic, hummus, salt, and pepper with water in a mixing bowl. Add the walnuts, olive, and dried cranberries, if desired. Set aside.

Add the pasta in the boiling water. Cook the pasta following the manufacturer's specifications until attaining an al dente texture. Drain the pasta.

4.Transfer the pasta to a large serving bowl and combine with the sauce.

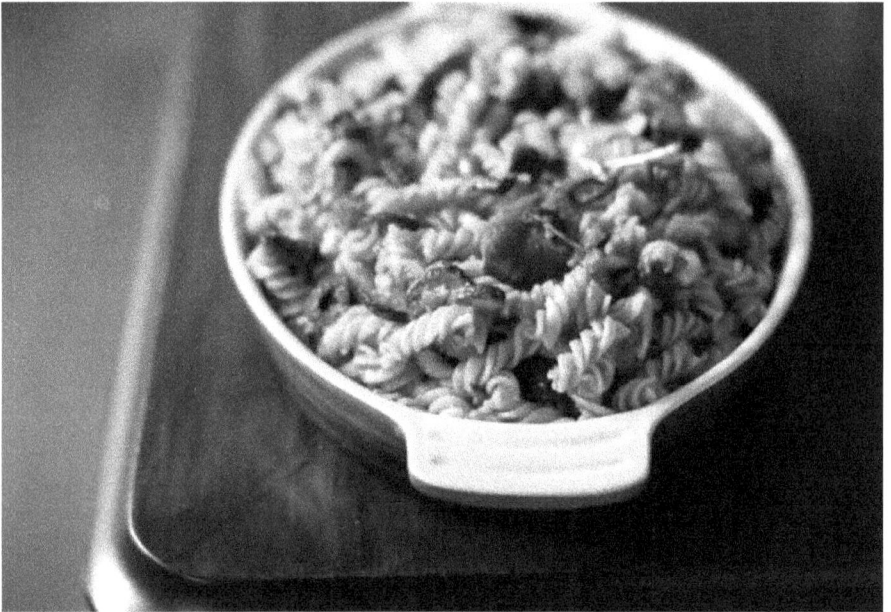

Cheesy Spaghetti with Pine Nuts

Preparation Time: 10 minutes

Cooking Time: 10 minutes

Servings: 4

Ingredients:
8 oz. spaghetti
4 tbsp. (½ stick) unsalted butter
1 tsp. freshly ground black pepper
½ cup pine nuts
1 cup fresh grated Parmesan cheese, divided

Directions:

1.Bring a large pot of salted water to a boil. Add the pasta and cook for 8 minutes.

2.In a large saucepan over medium heat, combine the butter, black pepper, and pine nuts. Cook for 2 to 3 minutes or until the pine nuts are lightly toasted.

Reserve ½ cup of the pasta water. Drain the pasta and put it into the pan with the pine nuts.

4.Add ¾ cup of Parmesan cheese and the reserved pasta water to the pasta and toss everything together to evenly coat it.

5.To serve, put the pasta in a serving dish and top with the remaining ¼ cup of Parmesan cheese.

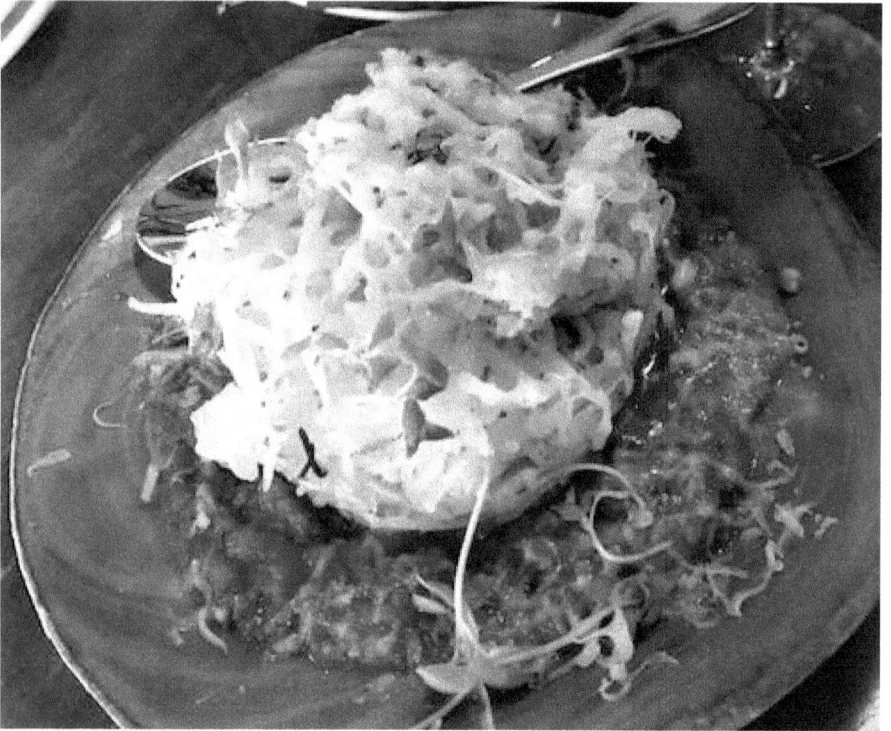

Fragrant Basmati Rice

Preparation Time: 5 minutes
Cooking Time: 17 minutes
Servings: 6

Ingredients:

1 cup long-grain rice
1 tbsp. olive oil
1 tsp. dried rosemary
    2 ½ cup water

Directions

1.Heat the olive oil in the saucepan.

2.Add rice and roast it for 2 minutes. Stir it constantly.

3.Then add rosemary and water.

4.Stir the rice and close the lid.

5.Cook it for 15 minutes or until it soaks all water.

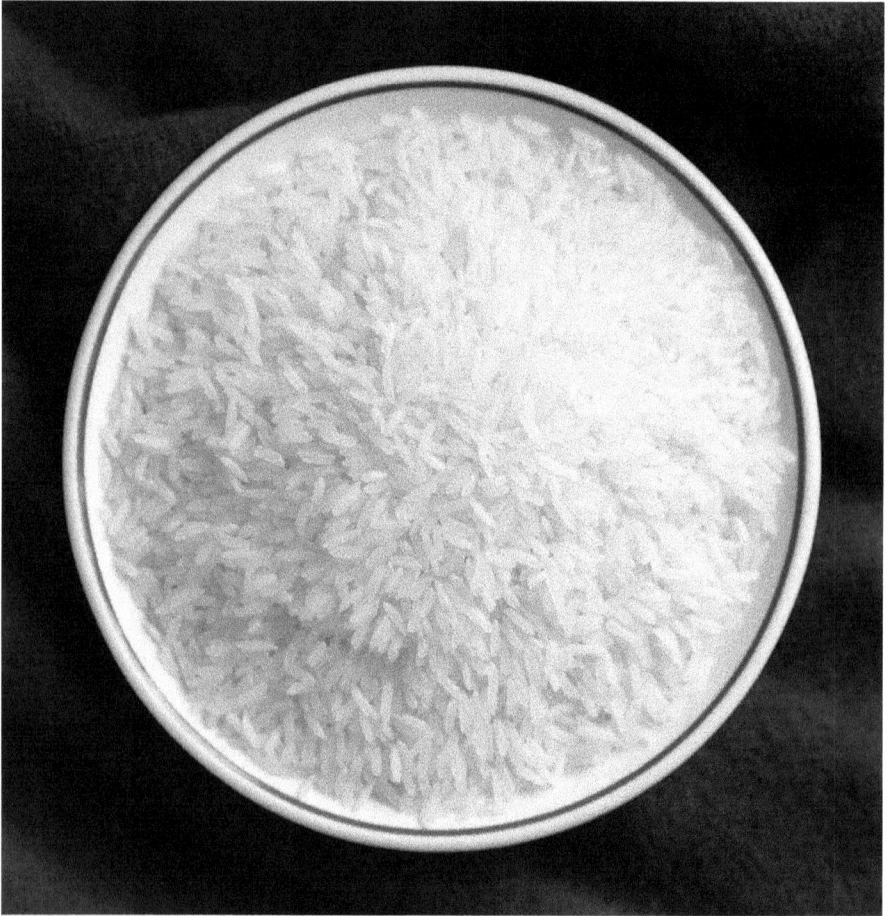

Cranberry Rice

Preparation Time: 5 minutes
Cooking Time: 20 minutes
Servings: 4

Ingredients:

¼ cup basmati rice
1 cup of organic almond milk
2 oz dried cranberries
¼ tsp. ground cinnamon

Directions:

1.Put all ingredients in the saucepan, stir, and close the lid.

2. Cook the rice on low heat for 20 minutes.

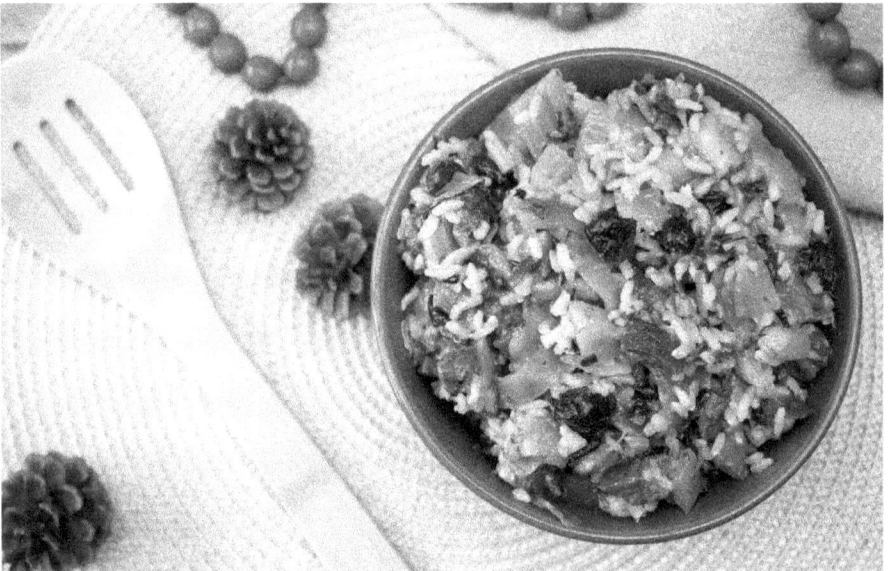

Brown Rice Saute

Preparation Time: 5 minutes

Cooking Time: 20 minutes

Servings: 3

Ingredients:

3 oz brown rice
9 oz chicken stock
1 tsp. curry powder
1 onion, diced
4 tbsp. olive oil

Directions:

1.Heat olive oil in the saucepan.

2.Add onion and cook it until light brown.

3.Add brown rice, curry powder, and chicken stock.

4.Close the lid and saute the rice for 15 minutes.

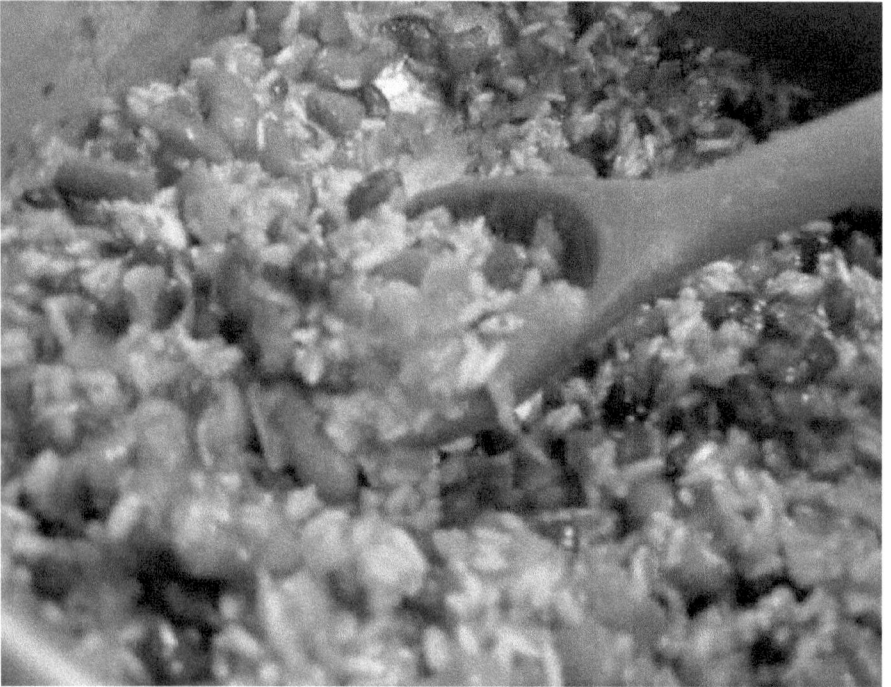

Pesto Rice

Preparation Time: 8 minutes

Cooking Time: 15 minutes

Servings: 4

Ingredients:

½ cup of basmati rice
1.5cup of water
2 tbsp. pesto sauce

Directions:

1. Simmer the rice water for 15 minutes on the low heat or until the rice soaks all liquid.

2.Then mix cooked tice with pesto sauce.

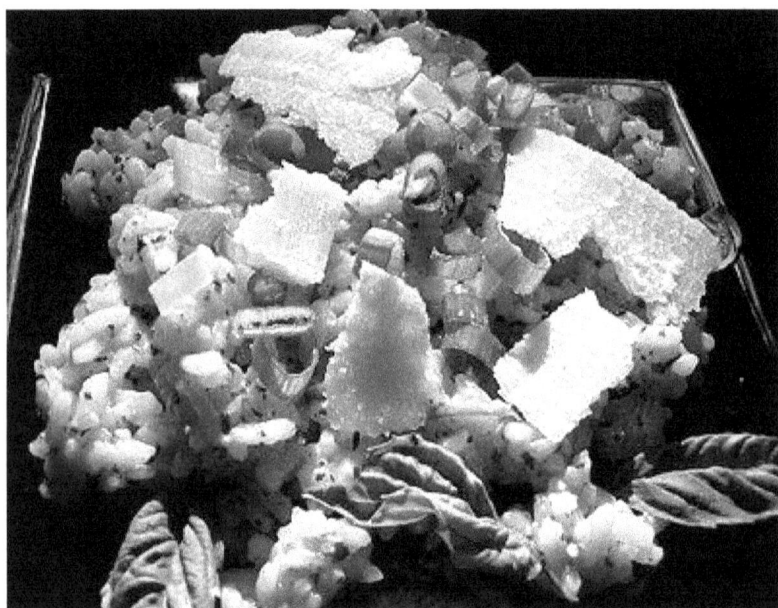

Rice Salad

Preparation Time: 10 minutes
Cooking Time: 0 minutes
Servings: 4

Ingredients:

½ cup long-grain rice, cooked
½ cup corn kernels, cooked 1 tomato, chopped
1 tsp. chili flakes
¼ cup plain yogurt 1 cucumber pickle

Directions:

1. Grate the cucumber pickle and mix it with cooked rice, corn kernels, tomato, chili flakes, and plain yogurt.

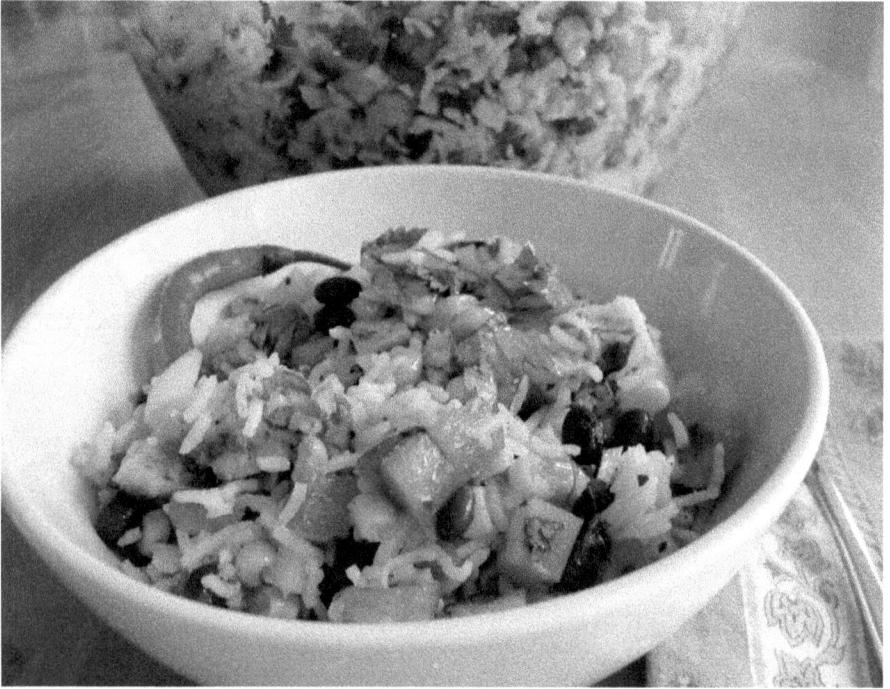

Rice Meatballs

Preparation Time: 10 minutes
Cooking Time: 15 minutes
Servings: 20

Ingredients:

¼ cup Cheddar cheese, shredded
1 tsp. ground black pepper
1 cup of basmati rice, cooked
¼ cup ground chicken
1 tsp. olive oil

Directions:

1.In the mixing bowl, mix Cheddar cheese, ground black pepper, rice, and ground chicken.

2.Then make the balls from the mixture.

3. Heat the olive oil well and put the rice balls in the hot oil.

4.Roast the balls for 1 minute per side on high heat.

5.Then transfer the balls in the oven and bake them for 20 minutes at 360F.

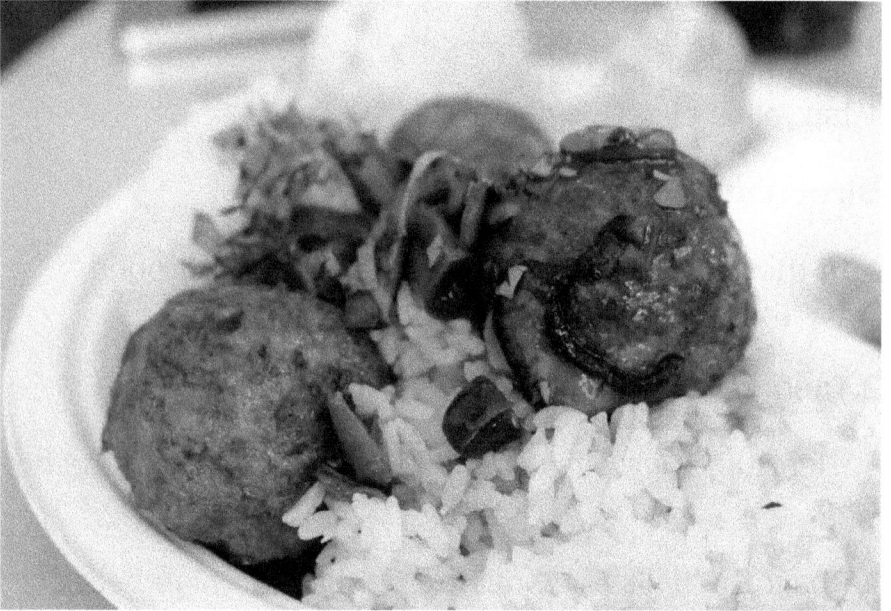

Mediterranean Paella

Preparation Time: 10 minutes
Cooking Time: 30 minutes
Servings: 6

Ingredients:

1 cup risotto rice
2 oz yellow onion, diced
½ tsp. ground paprika
1 cup tomatoes, chopped
1 cup shrimps, peeled
1 tsp. olive oil
3 cups of water

Directions:

1. Heat olive oil in the saucepan.

2.Add onion and cook it for 2 minutes.

3.Then stir well, add shrimps, ground paprika, tomatoes, and stir well.

4.Cook the ingredients for 5 minutes.

5.Add water and risotto rice. Stir well, close the lid, and cook the meal for 20 minutes on low heat.

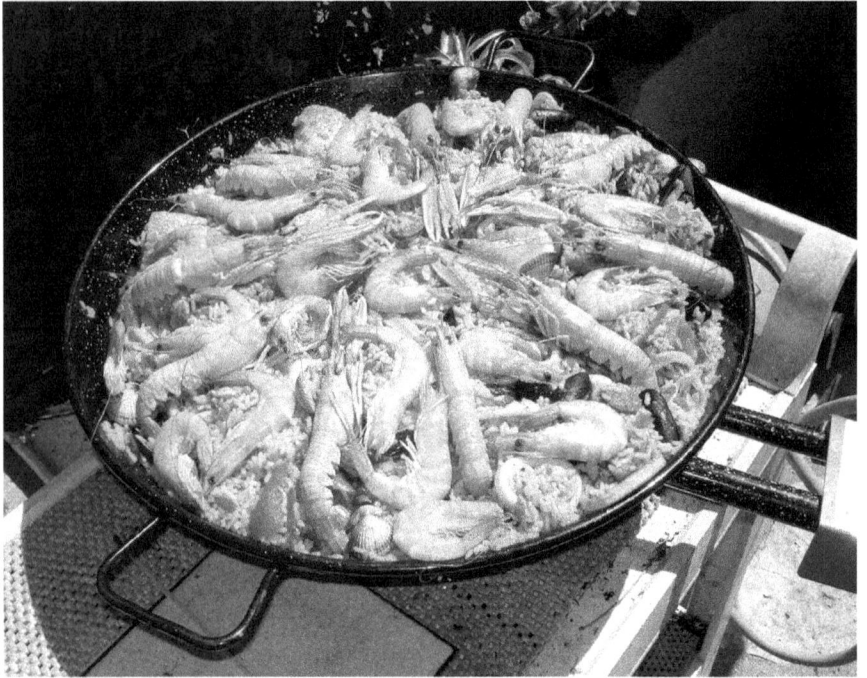

Fast Chicken

Rice Preparation Time: 10 minutes
Cooking Time: 20 minutes
Servings: 5

Ingredients:

1 cup basmati rice
3 tbsp. avocado oil
2.5cups chicken stock
½ tsp. dried dill
10 oz chicken breast, skinless, boneless, chopped

Directions:

1.Mix oil with rice and roast it in the saucepan for 5 minutes over the low heat.

2.Then add chicken and chicken stock.

3.Add dill, stir the ingredients and cook the meal on medium heat for 15 minutes or until all ingredients are cooked.

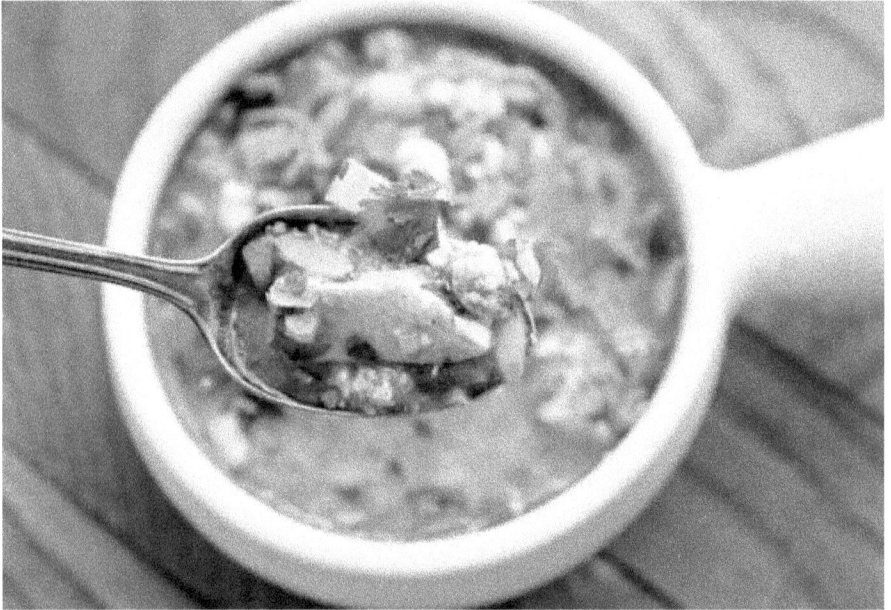

www.ingramcontent.com/pod-product-compliance
Lightning Source LLC
Chambersburg PA
CBHW050759030426
42336CB00012B/1877